TECHNIQUES OF CHILD THERAPY

TECHNIQUES OF CHILD THERAPY

Psychodynamic Strategies

SECOND EDITION

Morton Chethik

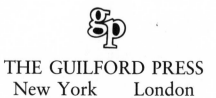

THE GUILFORD PRESS
New York   London

© 2000 The Guilford Press
A Division of Guilford Publications, Inc.
72 Spring Street, New York, NY 10012
www.guilford.com

Printed in the United States of America

This book is printed on acid-free paper.

Last digit is print number: 9 8 7 6 5 4 3 2

Library of Congress Cataloging-in-Publication Data

Chethik, Morton.
    Techniques of child therapy: psychodynamic strategies / Morton
Chethik.—2nd ed.
        p. cm.
    Includes bibliographical references and index.
    ISBN 1-57230-528-2 (cloth)   ISBN 1-57230-925-3 (paper)
        1. Child psychotherapy.   I. Title.
RJ504 .C463 2000
618.92′8914—dc21   00-034730

About the Author

MORTON CHETHIK is currently an emeritus professor in the Department of Psychiatry at the University of Michigan. He is Director of the Child Psychotherapy Program at the Michigan Psychoanalytic Society and continues his private practice in Ann Arbor, Michigan. A current area of his writing focuses on the special perspective that child therapy provides for understanding work with adult patients.

Preface

This, the second edition of *Techniques of Child Therapy*, remains oriented to both students (fellows in child psychiatry, clinical psychology interns, social work students) and more advanced practitioners in these mental health disciplines who are interested in sharpening their skills in child psychotherapy.

A number of cases were discussed in the first edition. The major reason for the revision was to markedly expand this focus and elaborate on the *specifics of the clinical process with children and parents* in a step-by-step presentation. Two major case write-ups are added detailing the process from intake through termination, sharing my ideas and reactions throughout the cases, and further highlighting the specifics of techniques that are difficult to spell out in condensed case reports.

Another area of revision is related to our understanding of the role of *play* in child therapy. Although play was discussed in the first edition, in the past 10 years there has been a substantial body of thought presented in the literature about play in development, its use in the therapeutic hour, and its enhancement of the alliance between child and therapist. These ideas are fully reviewed and clinically illustrated in a new presentation in Chapter 3, "The Central Role of Play." Understanding the function of play is critical for the child practitioner.

This book retains the basic definitions and concepts of psychotherapy described in the first edition as well as the discussion and illustration of varied child psychpathologies. It also retains and further illustrates the assessment process and the varied approaches to work with parents, allowing the reader to move easily between clinical theory and clinical cases within a single expanded work.

Contents

TECHNIQUES OF CHILD THERAPY

I

~

Introduction to Child Therapy

Introduction

The purpose of this part of the book is to introduce the reader to the child as a young patient. This means becoming familiar with the emotional and cognitive world of the child and contrasting his readiness for psychotherapy with that of the older patient (the adult). Chapters 1 and 3 focus on these differences. Some of the divergences stem from the child's "immaturity," his dependency on his parents, and the fact that he is in an ongoing developmental process. These differences alter the process of the therapy, its format, and, at times, the goals of the treatment itself. The material in this part of the book illustrates and discusses the necessary revisions.

An essential modification in work with children, as compared with adults, is the basic form of communication between patient and therapist. A primary purpose of all psychotherapy is to work with the patient's affective life. Play becomes a central medium of exchange with most children, as this is the child's major mode of expressing his emotional life. Chapter 3 introduces the reader to this medium. It focuses on how important play is in development, in adulthood as well as in childhood. The chapter describes how to set the stage to play, how to facilitate its development in the treatment hour, and how to use it when it emerges. These themes are followed throughout the course of the book, embedded in the clinical material.

Whereas Chapters 1 and 3 serve as a general introduction to the process of child treatment, the evaluation process in any given case alerts the therapist to the issues and problems that will emerge in a specific child's treatment. The evaluation "introduces" the therapy itself. Chapter 2 discusses how to conduct an evaluation, how to construct a psychodynamic formulation, and how an effective personality appraisal can be used to outline, anticipate, and enhance the therapeutic process.

1

~

General Characteristics of the Child Patient

Before one attempts child psychotherapy, it is imperative to become oriented to the state of childhood and to the world of the child. The purpose of this chapter is to "set the stage" and provide a general orientation to the young patient. A common, unfortunate tendency is to carry the adult world and an adult model of treatment into child therapy. In adult psychotherapy, most treatment techniques have been developed for dealing with a patient with a relatively stabilized, structured personality and ego. The hallmark of the child patient, however, is that his personality is in a state of evolution and flux, and his ego is immature. What does it mean to attempt therapy when defenses are naturally fragile, when cognitive capacity is poor, when anxiety is easily stimulated, when superego is limited, and when magic and omnipotence can prevail? In this chapter, five major issues are discussed:

1. *The fluctuating state of the child's ego.* The child's ego is fragile and undeveloped, making him/her a very different kind of patient.
2. *The child's need for action: the function of play.* Action dominates in child's work, and the therapist must become a player.
3. *The child's state of dependency: the role of the parents.* A

major task is understanding and often modifying the family dynamics.

4. *The child's developmental process: the need for growth.* The treatment relationship includes the therapist as a real object, a figure for identification, and as "developmental facilitator."

5. *The counterreactions to the child patient: the therapist's internal reactions.* The child patient evokes unique emotional "wear and tear" responses that are essential to understand.

THE FLUCTUATING STATE OF THE CHILD'S EGO

The child's ego, by the nature of development, is a fluid one as compared with that of the adult; it is constantly shifting and regressing and is much closer to the world of primary process. Often, a fluidity of ego boundaries exists, particularly during periods of stress. By *primary process*, we mean that there is a suspension or lack of the logical part of the mind, and the elements of the unconscious are expressed in primitive forms with no awareness of time present. With few exceptions, then, *acting out* dominates in the treatment of the child. He tends to live out his pleasures and anxieties and shows his disorders in the form of direct action and play (Olden, 1953; Freud, 1965; Anthony, 1964). Davies (1999) discusses some of the specific anxieties in childhood that create disruptive behavior: reactions to aggressive feelings, fears of being displaced in the parents' affections, failures in the control of bodily functions, fear and distress about being rejected by peers, fears caused by inadequate reality testing and magical thinking.

To address this issue, it may be helpful to consider a young child patient. Mark, a 5½-year-old youngster, in the course of his evaluation and early treatment, vividly highlights the state of childhood. His affect state was quite volatile. Although Mark was clearly a disturbed youngster, he nonetheless illustrates, albeit sometimes in an exaggerated way, all of the issues that arise in working with the child patient.

Clinical Material

Mark was referred because of his long-standing defiant fighting and his frequently out-of-control behavior. Mark was a rather short but well-built, well-proportioned child who looked "ready for action." He was pleasant looking with striking dark features and coloring, resembling his mother. He appeared extremely restless. One found Mark climbing, twisting, or hurtling rather than walking from place to place.

His parents described the fighting relationship Mark had with others, particularly with his mother, and they noted they were at their "wits' end" in their attempts to handle him. They felt they had exhausted all possible methods—they had talked with Mark, reasoned with him, punished and spanked, and had even given him a special half hour of "Mark time" per day, but nothing had seemed to work.

In the history, the difficulties with Mark seemed to begin during his second year, when his mother was pregnant with his brother Richard. (There were three boys in the family: Jason was 2 years older than Mark, and Richard was 2 years younger.) The summer during this pregnancy had been particularly hot and humid, and Mrs. L found that carrying Richard was difficult and tiring. Mark was a very active toddler. In addition, she was aware of a change within herself. She became more easily angered with him and had less patience. She had told the boys about her impending delivery the night before Richard was born, and Mark had begun climbing out of his crib.

When Mrs. L returned home with the new baby, the difficulties began to compound. One evening she found Mark straddling the baby in his crib, and she then began to lock Mark in his room at night. Because of his vigorous protest, she recanted and opened the door. But Mark was now incessantly climbing out of his crib. She and her husband, in an effort to keep him in bed, built higher and higher barriers on his crib side. Showing incredible effort, Mark scaled all the obstacles in order to get free.

This defiant pattern carried over into all areas of the family's life. With toilet training, Mark would be forced to sit on the potty but would soil right after he got off. The mother would become angered and lose her temper. Mark was "trained" at 3 years of age for bowel and bladder, although at the point of evaluation he was enuretic nightly, soiled from time to time, and wet himself occasionally during the day. The mother also described a pattern of provocative soiling—at times he would simply pull down his pants and defecate on a neighbor's lawn.

As his horizons broadened, Mark's antisocial behavior spread. He became somewhat of a "terror" in the community. He was often aggressive with street friends; he would suddenly hit and punch without provocation. He would lead little forays into neighbors' yards and might turn on a hose and have the water flow into the kitchen or basement. His mother noted sarcastically that the family had become "real popular" on the block.

Despite the history of behavior difficulty and out-of-control action, it was impossible to anticipate completely the furor of the first few months of treatment. Mark was often totally out of control after the first few minutes of each interview. His behavior seemed to evidence panic, aggression, and self-destruction. An example of an early session follows.

Mark entered the office and quickly ran to the house and block toys. Within a few moments he created a mommy bed and a daddy bed in one room, a baby bed in the other. A tremendous fight ensued between the mommy and daddy beds, with the daddy getting on top often. Frightening noises emerged from the room, and the baby was scared.

Suddenly the blocks flew and the house was overturned. Quickly Mark began climbing on the furniture, heedless of anything the therapist might say; he jumped and threw himself on the couch until he hurt his arm. He cried out in pain and then rested for a few minutes. Suddenly he was off again. Now he decided to take off his shoes and socks and rip a hole in his pants. He seemed to be in a frenzy, overturning all chairs, throwing the pillows, and yelling at the therapist. He appeared terribly frightened and called out for his mother, whom Mark and the therapist then visited. He ended the interview by pulling down his pants and attempting to urinate on the floor. It seemed that any game or play that Mark turned to quickly brought forth material that had enormous anxieties attached to it. The previously described primal-scene material was only one example. Children typically express anxiety by motoric discharge. Thus, when Mark became anxious about the sexual material his play uncovered, he expressed his anxiety in the language of children—through yelling, throwing, and fighting.

After 2 weeks of treatment, his parents reported in an "emergency" appointment that Mark had attacked another boy so badly (dragged him by the hood of his jacket for a full block) that he had to be accompanied to and from school. The principal had warned them that this incident, together with Mark's history of difficulties, might mean that Mark would be suspended from school.

It soon became clear that the therapist needed to establish firm and rigid controls. At the first sign of trouble, the therapist emptied all "throwables" from the room—chairs, pillows, papers all went into the closet, which was closed for the rest of that hour. The climbing rules (e.g., going onto the table or couch with shoes is not allowed) had to be absolutely enforced, with no second chances given. The therapist escorted Mark to the bathroom and would enter at any point if needed. Throughout this early treatment period of establishing a safe surround and structure, the therapist worked verbally and behaviorally on differentiating between control and punishment. For example, in the early treatment period the therapist sometimes needed to hold Mark. Mark would, at times, look terrified, as if he expected to be hurt. The therapist then quietly explained that he held Mark so he would not break anything or hurt himself and that he would let him go as soon as Mark was calmer. Later, when things were calm, he would further discuss why he held him, even though Mark worried that the therapist would hurt him.

The openness of the therapy situation quickly brought forth in Mark internal material that was terrifying (e.g., the mommy and daddy beds), and the therapist noted the regression, terror, and disorder. Anthony (1982) has described the young child in cognitive terms:

> The child, as Piaget was the first to point out, is dominated by egocentrism. He is not a self-conscious thinker, and he differs radically from the adolescent or the adult. His mind is essentially concrete, simplistically operational, and committed to the present. The child never thinks about what he is thinking about, has limited powers of reflection and has difficulties in making spontaneous associations between ideas and events widely separated in time and space.

This relatively undeveloped state of the child's ego has implications at the start of the treatment process.

Capacity for Motivation

Whereas the child lacks the fundamental capacity for motivation at the start of treatment (Tyson & Tyson, 1986), the potential adult patient has many different capacities. Initially, the adult reviews his current emotional life and becomes aware of important failings. For example, he may acknowledge that he has repeated difficulties in making effective sexual relationships and conclude that somehow he is contributing to his own problems. Or he may recognize that he consistently falls short in his work efforts even though he is bright. He imagines a future state in which he is symptom-free and can prosper both with the opposite sex and in his work life. The new ingredient that potentially can promote this change is psychotherapy, whereby he can shed his inhibitions and resistances. Thus, the adult patient has a number of ego capacities, including a *self-observing capacity* to view the state of the self and a capacity to *project himself into the future* to view an enhanced state. These capacities are not at all available to the child patient (Rees, 1978). In the early sessions described previously, Mark clearly wanted to run away from this new and frightening situation. The therapeutic environment was a scary place, and he participated only because he was forced by his family. His attitude is typical of children, and we do not see the motivation that is evident in the adult patient.

It is interesting to note, however, that Mark did express affective material in an early session, where the mommy bed and daddy bed (sexual activity) scare the baby bed. Mark did not consciously bring the material as a communication to the therapy. The underlying instinctual material emerges in the play and action of the child, and it serves as a directional force in the child's treatment. However, it would be misleading to suggest that the child "brings" this material to the therapy as a participant.

Capacity to Tolerate Pain and Anxiety

Mark, like most children, cannot sustain the idea that he has a problem at all, and thus he differs from the adult patient. Part of the capacity to acknowledge an internal problem depends on the ability to tolerate a modicum of anxiety and discomfort. Children have an enormous tendency to *externalize* all problems and shift the blame outside (Bornstein, 1948). For example, when the therapist noted that Mark perhaps had a "fighting problem" in school, Mark immediately justified his behavior with his classmates. He *knew* that they were *all* angry with him and they all wanted to beat him up. Confrontations of logic like "You mean, everybody in your class wants to beat you up?" made no inroads into his need to project blame from himself and avoid the unpleasant situation. The child patient like Mark is not an eager participant in the early stages of treatment.

The Therapist as a Frightening Object

The description of a "talking, helping person" related to Mark by his parents was seen by Mark as an attempt to lull him from his fears about the dangers in this new strange surround. He reacted with terror and attacks. His clear wish was to get away from this anxiety-producing situation and flee from treatment. Children have little capacity to establish an early alliance. Many beginning child therapists see themselves as wanting to be helpful and caring toward the child patient. The child's image of the therapist rarely corresponds with the therapist's image.

In summary, children are rarely motivated initially, typically seek flight from an anxiety-producing situation, and project (ascribe their own internal feelings to a person outside) the aggression and attacking motivations they are encountering to the therapist. The child's ego state usually makes him an unwilling patient. Generally, in child work one has to respect the vulnerability of the child's immature ego. One needs to be aware of the degree of frustration a child can tolerate and must be attuned to the child's feeling state (Harley, 1986). Building an alliance and helping children to become aware of their internal difficulties is a task for the therapist in the early part of the treatment.

THE CHILD'S NEED FOR ACTION: THE FUNCTION OF PLAY

In adult psychotherapy, the basic method of transmitting the patient's affective life is through verbalization. Children, however, are in the process of developing their secondary process thinking functions as well as their capacity for symbol formation. Verbalization, therefore, is difficult, particularly for affective expression (Peller, 1954). The natural tendency for the child is bodily discharge for all discomfort and tension, as Mark portrayed.

Children do learn the "language" of the adult world and often use it for its propaganda value. Thus, Mark told his therapist early in their encounters that he came to see him for his "fighting problems." This was not a piece of self-observation but rather a palliative thrown to the therapist to keep him at bay. Mark did not feel that his fighting was a problem at all—indeed, for him it was a necessary form of survival in a projected hostile world.

Children naturally develop their affective world and express it developmentally in active, partly verbal form—*play* (Sandler, Kennedy, & Tyson, 1980). Play emerges from the child's internal life and typically explicates major conflicts or defenses. When a 6-year-old puts on two six-shooters and a sheriff's badge and struts through the household, he is often attempting to deal with a natural internal source of helplessness and smallness. He temporarily masters his sense of littleness in fantasy, and he makes use of this process, in varied forms, throughout his childhood. As Anthony (1986) points out, "young patients talk more freely, spontaneously and less defensively in the language of play since they seem to regard this special realm, preconsciously, as once removed from the pressures and demands of everyday life."

The child therapist needs to capitalize on this form of communication, which is "in between" primitive behavior and verbalization. In fact, the therapist's office should be a "playground" so that the child's world can be projected—an unstructured setting that has paper, crayons, scissors, blocks, dolls, and so forth, where the child's internal characters can come to life. The task of the therapist is to facilitate the emergence of the child's stories. The following clinical material shows the development of play in the early stages of Mark's treatment.

Clinical Material

Mark's early extreme behavior in treatment expressed a fusion of many fears, but slowly certain themes became discernible and therefore more easily handled. Mark was terrified of the office, terrified of the therapist, and frightened of the separation from his mother during his sessions. Through his behavior rather than words, Mark revealed that he was worried about the overhead light, the holes in the soundproofing, the closet, and its door. The therapist began a vigorously active game with Mark. This was a critical juncture. The therapist, using the fears that Mark expressed, put them into play form. The therapist announced a game called "torture chamber," verbalizing Mark's fearful appraisal of the office, and the closet became the "torture chamber." With that introduction, Mark led the action. Either he or the therapist was locked in for days. They were beaten or starved or left without any water to drink. Mark cried and wailed. Only after this game had been repeated many times did direct words make any sense. The therapist could then proclaim: "No wonder you are hitting and kicking, if you thought this could happen to you here."

Alternatively, Mark decided to play "living room." He knocked and entered the "living room," not the office. He sat down comfortably and ordered food and milk to drink, which the therapist gave in play. The office became home, the therapist became the giving mother, and Mark induced the game when worried about separation.

After about a month of treatment, Mark was using more play. The themes were often danger, attack, counterattack, and victory. For example, the pillow became a monster that suddenly leapt on him. At first he was overwhelmed, but then, as a growling monster himself, he overcame the adversary. As a growling monster, however, he might go on to stalk the furniture and the therapist. The therapist began to identify the growling out-of-control part of Mark as the "lion part." "When you become scared, you become the lion." "There, we see the lion again." "How much does the wild lion part of Mark get him into trouble?" "He never knows what the lion will do—how it will suddenly come out." Mark's behavior was often impulsive. One day he smashed a favorite Etch-a-Sketch toy he had brought to show his therapist because he was proud of his design production. The therapist could identify with Mark's own shock and surprise after the lion erupted. "What is going to happen to Mark?" the therapist wondered with him.

The lion part of Mark also did not heed the normal rules of caution and safety, and it had a daredevil quality. Mark brought a Mighty Mouse doll into the therapy, which he related he slept with. In the sessions, Mighty Mouse sat precariously at the edge of the windowsill and, with Mark's help, tottered into the chasm below. Or Mighty Mouse was perched on the top of the play table. A wind hurled him onto boulders in the valley below, but at the last moment, Mighty Mouse flew off unharmed—he was invulnerable.

A problem in Mark's general behavior was his need to flirt with danger. His mother had reported his practice of riding his two-wheeler at full speed on the streets without looking for cars. The daredevil wandered off several times, crossing heavy traffic. One day the therapist received a call that Mark had climbed out onto the roof, which had a steep incline, in the rain. At first, when the therapist introduced some of these incidents in a quiet and serious vein, Mark evidenced bravado. But with the roof incident, when the therapist noted that the lion part of Mark might one day take him too far and that something could happen that he could never change or make good again, Mark evinced an overpowering fear reaction. He was suddenly exhausted, lay on the couch sucking his thumb, stroking his ear, and holding onto his penis. He told the therapist that maybe he could fall off and die.

The lion part of Mark was becoming more ego-alien. In one session, after a strong tussle with his therapist, Mark became reflective. He told his therapist that it was very hard for him to be good. The therapist acknowledged that it was a problem but felt he could help Mark with it. Mark began a series of confessions, which he played out in games. He told his therapist of a boy named Gary, not Mark, who was very wild but afraid of ghosts. Mark made it "night" in the office (darkened the room) and reenacted scenes. A robber came to steal his money, and Gary was scared. Even when the robber was jailed, he repeatedly escaped to scare the boy again. When the therapist noted that Mark himself was scared every night and seemed to have bad dreams, Mark wanted to know if the therapist "could take them away."

In addition, Mark began to examine all parts of his body for sores and scratches and acknowledged worries about things being broken. The problem of soiling was played out. One day the therapist and Mark took a make-believe ride on a train (two chairs next to one another), and suddenly Mark made "doo" in his pants. He took out the pretend "doo," threw it in the therapist's face, and told him he was so ugly he couldn't look at him. When the therapist noted that it must be hard for him in school when Mark sometimes "makes doo" in his class, Mark said very sadly that his name was "Underwear" in the classroom, and "You know what that means—dirty underwear."

Mark's behavior in the office now changed dramatically. At times he could discuss some fears and show his anxieties, yet while sucking his thumb. He could also become totally absorbed in productive craftwork, in which he had many skills. He drew at length and constructed involved castles replete with moats, turrets, and interesting walls out of Legos and blocks.

The therapeutic alliance began to emerge in a more mature form as Mark shifted from sheer action to some focus on inner concerns and worries.

In the preceding clinical case material, the therapist initially worked carefully to make a bridge between the child patient's out-of-control behavior and play. He picked up on Mark's fears and terrors by inventing a "torture chamber" game as Mark looked furtively at the closet. As this game was played out, Mark's anxiety began to take a coherent form that both therapist and patient could observe. Only then could the therapist's verbalization be integrated—"No wonder you are hitting and kicking, if you thought this could happen to you here." One of the major functions of play is to alter the raw, overwhelming affects that arise in children at times of anxiety and provide a natural vehicle for the expression of these affects.

Because play emerges from the child's internal life, it typically explicates major internal issues. After a short period of treatment, Mark introduced Mighty Mouse. Mighty Mouse faced all sorts of terrible catastrophies, from which he escaped at the last moment. For example, blown off a mountain and about to smash into a deep chasm, Mighty Mouse used his magic capacity to fly just in the nick of time. Mighty Mouse was clearly a self-representation; that is, he depicted Mark. Mark himself was little and always frightened that the grown-up world would attack him—he had many fears of annihilation and castration. He, like Mighty Mouse, faced or provoked dangers, which he "fearlessly" confronted and then used magical means to escape. Should the real Mark become frightened of the cars on the street, he would "fearlessly" drive his two-wheel bicycle into the middle of traffic, defying any danger. Mighty Mouse in his play depicted Mark who in this case had developed a counterphobic character style to deal with enormous internal anxiety. The task of the child therapist is to provide the structure to facilitate the emergence of these internal characters, so that patient and therapist can slowly think about them together.

The therapist needs not only to set the scene for play, but also to become a "player" in the child's world. As Mark attacked the therapist and growled, the therapist played out roles under Mark's direction. Therapist and child played out the growling monster and the frightened man. At the same time, using words the child could understand, the therapist moved toward the goal of verbalization. The therapist sought to have Mark identify a part of himself—his "lion part." This technique promoted Mark's self-observation in nonjudgmental manner (lions can attack and fight at times, but they are also brave). Later Mark and his therapist together could determine what triggered the lion and got him into trouble. The therapist could begin to work with Mark to determine the cause and effect of his aggression, but this interchange could occur meaningfully only through the child's play world. This theory is more fully examined in a later chapter (Chapter 3) and throughout the text.

This period of work with Mark saw a change and a developing alliance with the therapist. Mark expressed genuine concern about his behavior ("It's hard for me to be a good boy") and evidenced his frightening dreams, his anxiety about scratches, his "doo" (soiling) problem. He looked to the therapist to remove these bad worries.

After a period of time in therapy, it is often possible to help the young patient to give up some of his need for externalization (expelling the problem outside and denying his involvement). Several factors can foster greater internal awareness. One is the therapist's general stance of confronting problematic behavior in an accepting, nonjudgmental way. For example, at issue was Mark's fighting difficulties. When the therapist highlighted these difficulties as Mark's "lion feelings," they could be explored without Mark's anxiety that he was being attacked. He was proud of his strength, although there were times it got him into trouble. A second factor is that of identification. As a positive attachment develops, the young patient will want to identify with the therapist. Often the therapist will encourage secondary process thinking (the mature modes of reason, verbalization, etc.). Thus, Mark's therapist could emphasize how well Mark was using his "thinker" at times or convey how impressed he was when Mark could listen to the therapist this time even though it made him scared.

THE CHILD'S STATE OF DEPENDENCY: THE ROLE OF THE PARENTS

Another major difference that powerfully affects the process of therapy with the child is the child's marked physical and emotional dependency on his family. The child is exceedingly close to his parents, and his parents provide the major source of motivation for growth and development—the major sources of pleasures as well as fears. The need for object love and approval and the fear of object loss both shape the course of the development of the child's drives (what impulses are acceptable), ego capacities (through identification), and superego formation (internalization of parental prohibitions and values), (Ackerman, 1958; Cutter & Hallowitz, 1982; Fraiberg, 1954; Kessler, 1966). Davies (1999) cites a number of "parental risk factors" like high parental conflict, family disruption, harsh parenting, coercive family process, and child maltreatment that markedly effects the growing child. Understanding the parent–child relationship must be a central part of the diagnostic process, and when necessary, modifying the problems in the parent–child relationship must be a part of the child treatment process.

In recent years, there has been a good deal of social science research on the object tie between parent and child using Bowlby's (1988) attachment theories. Essentially insecure adults become insecure parents and quickly develop disturbances in their offspring. Distinctive patterns emerge in these population samples. "Dismissive" parents are likely to develop "Avoidant" infants (Main et al., 1985). "Preoccupied" adults develop "Ambivalent" infants (Bartholomew & Horowitz, 1991), and "Disorganized" parents tend to produce "Disoriented" infants (Main & Hesse, 1990). These findings corroborate the idea that parents have an enormous influence on the emotional development of their children.

In the treatment situation, a good working alliance with the child's parents is critical, because the child will be very much aware of the parental attitude toward the treatment. Ritvo (1978) pointed out that "just as the parent invests the toy for the young child in the interest of play, so the adult invests the therapist for the child in the interest of the relief of discomfort and suffering."

Unfortunately, the work with parents is often resisted or seen as an enormous encumbrance. Several authors openly advocate little or no contact, whereas others reluctantly shoulder the "burden" (Kohrman, Fineberg, Gelman, & Weiss, 1971). It is my opinion that parent work is an absolutely central aspect of child therapy and that most cases succeed or fail based on the quality of that aspect of the work. The following material highlights Mark's interaction with his mother.

Clinical Material

It was clear from Mark's history that there was a long-standing adversarial relationship between mother and son. In the weekly meetings with Mark's mother, Mrs. L was extremely cooperative and consciously and quickly (on advice) established more effective limits in the home, which helped to begin to control Mark's acting out. When we came to understand that some of Mark's chaos sprang from intense excitements, Mrs. L (on the home front) established privacy in the bathroom and curtailed Mark's visits to her bedroom when she dressed.

After several months of treatment, the daredevil theme became prominent in Mark's behavior. In the office, he climbed extensively; it was as if he were challenged by an obstacle and sought to master it. For instance, it became important for him to determine whether he could climb to the high windowsill and sit there. But the desire for danger was never mastered. He next wanted to see whether he could move across the windowsill, and when that was accomplished, he attempted to do it in a standing position, and on and on. Slowly, it became evident that Mark's mother played an important part in this counterphobic method of handling danger.

In a session, his mother related that Mark, a nonswimmer, had wandered off to the neighborhood pool. The family had been terribly worried for a number of hours, but as she told of the frightening event, a characteristic smile of pure pleasure illuminated her face. Mark was fantastically resourceful: He found the pool himself seven blocks from home; he persuaded the guard to allow him to enter, despite the rules that he needed a parent and that he was well under 48 inches, the minimum height for admission. (In his therapy at this point, Mark was preoccupied with fears of drowning.) His mother related all such events, all difficult situations and narrow escapes that Mark was involved in, as high adventures and gave clear indications of an underlying intense pleasure. It was apparent that a good deal of Mark's frightening chance taking was libidinally reinforced by Mrs. L. She subtly conveyed her pleasure to him. She was aware and accepted that although Mark's escapades frightened her, they also provided a part of her with some pleasure. These reactions became an area of our work together.

Throughout the contacts with Mrs. L, the therapist was impressed by her special identification with Mark. Although Mark might be more disturbed than his two brothers, she pointed out, he also had unique potentials. He was brighter than they were, he had a special tenacity the others did not have, and he was the most physically attractive child. She could always get the older brother, Jason, to do what she wanted; he would dress himself without question with the clothing she laid out for him. But if Mark determined he wanted to wear something of his own choosing, she could stand on her head and it would make no difference. As she related these incidents, her characteristic smile conveyed the obvious pleasure at the manly aggressiveness that Mark displayed.

Mrs. L's special tie to Mark had started early. When he was born, she had felt that he was particularly attractive partly because he was completely covered with hair. The family joke was that they would leave the hospital to go directly to the barbershop. In addition, when Mrs. L was a child, her hairiness was a family topic for years.

Mrs. L had been a happy child, she felt, but had always had a difficult time with her own mother. In order to maintain a sense of identity, Mrs. L had had to fight her own mother every inch of the way. It was not that her mother had been mean, but she had always wanted to be the complete boss. Mrs. L recalled that when she was organizing her sweet 16 party her mother had tried to take over all the arrangements. When the daughter reacted, her mother had continued to interfere, and the girl moved the party to a friend's house where she could manage it completely by herself. This pattern of clear assertion continued even during Mrs. L's married life. Her mother would wonder whether she was keeping the dishes in the "right place," she had new suggestions for furniture arrangements, and so forth. Mrs. L would totally resist all ideas, as a result of which mother and daughter highly respected each other. This mutual esteem was in contrast to the relationship between her mother and her younger sister, who acted like a child and was very dependent on her mother.

With this history, Mrs. L could appreciate the therapist's interpretations that she cherished the feisty little Mark who would never be beaten down, inasmuch as he recalled and expressed her own feisty struggles with her mother. Part of her, of course, knew that Mark needed firm and authoritative limits, but another part inside her wanted to see Mark never knuckle down or be crushed by the authorities around him. As Mrs. L became increasingly aware that her limit setting would not choke the spirit out of Mark, she could effectively take command with less ambivalence. She could also, with skill, anticipate when Mark's "manly" defiance would promote her subtle pleasure, and the therapist found that she went far in mastering what affects she conveyed to Mark. They also worked on new areas in which Mark's tenacity and activity could be expressed appropriately.

In each specific child therapy, a major diagnostic need is a review of both past and current parent–child interactions. How do they interact, and in what ways, if any, does this interaction support the child's pathology? In Mark's case, on a conscious level Mrs. L was very supportive of treatment and able, with the therapist's aid, to set effective limits and control overt sexual stimulation. It became increasingly clear that on an unconscious level, the mother significantly reinforced Mark's daredevil and counterphobic tendencies. No therapeutic intervention with Mark alone could alter the pleasure he experienced in living out his mother's underlying wishes.

In this case, as in most child psychotherapies, the work with the parents was critical. The therapist helped the mother to become aware of their (mother–son) mutual pleasure, helped to make this source of gratification ego-alien, and helped the mother understand the internal emotional origins that fostered a repetition in her new family. Dealing with the parents' roles is essential in a child's case. Depending on the depth of influence, there are a hierarchy of techniques and various levels of intervention with parents available to the child therapist (Chethik, 1976). This subject is discussed in detail and illustrated particularly in the next section of the book.

THE CHILD'S DEVELOPMENTAL PROCESS: THE NEED FOR GROWTH

One of the major differences in child work is that the therapist has an additional important function that is not typically a part of adult psychotherapy. The child is in the process of development, and his presentation often expresses aspects of an ongoing developmental process. The therapist must not only work with the central conflicts that have brought the child to therapy but also deal with the manifestations and stresses of normal development that emerge (Curtis, 1979). Child therapists quickly become aware that the child patient is rapidly changing as he grows: His ego is expanding; his consciousness and self-consciousness are developing; he is tentatively establishing identities; and he develops a repertoire of defenses and coping skills (Anthony, 1982). Because new psychic structures are in the process of being formed, the therapist is in a central position to be instrumental in facilitating the child's developmental needs. Anna Freud (1965) noted that the therapist is also a "new and real object" to the child, inasmuch as the child has a hunger for all new experiences and relationships. It is primarily in slowly fostering the verbalization process that the therapist can help the child's ego to expand and master. The following clinical material discussed illustrates how the therapist helped Mark understand the typical sexual distortions all children develop, as well as those specific issues unique to Mark.

Clinical Material

Toward the end of the first year of treatment, Mark brought in a series of sexual fantasies over a period of months. He announced one day that he was not afraid of snakes and spiders: They were made out of chemicals. His father had many chemicals, and he wanted the therapist to know that his father made people from these chemicals, which he could mix from a stack in the basement. His father himself had been made in the hospital by hospital men. When his father had come home, he made his mother and, in turn, his three children in chronological order. Because Mark could only remember things from 4 years of age, he concluded that he had been made at the age of 4.

These ideas proved to be a prelude to action. In the next session Mark opened his fly, and the therapist was about to restrain him. However, Mark was very involved in a fantasy and not sexually aroused (also not exposed). He claimed he had many secret pockets inside his pants legs, and each pocket held a chemical. He "took out" certain chemicals and rubbed his hands in a very deliberate and systematic way. Suddenly he thrust his hands out—an explosion and fire took place, and babies were formed. The therapist and Mark found these babies in many places; they were heard crying in different parts of the room, and Mark took them out very tenderly.

The therapist then encroached in a number of ways: "Mark finds it hard sometimes to think that you need a mommy and daddy to have a baby." "Mark has a smart idea—there *are* special daddy chemicals that help make babies. We can think about that in the Body Book we're making." "Mark would really like to make babies, like his mommy."

Several weeks later, Mark was preoccupied with birth fantasies. At first he was interested in some universal elements, such as the differences between light and darkness. His thought was that the sun shone light during the day, and he concluded that the moon *shone* darkness at night (rather than perceiving that darkness was the absence of light). Thoughts of God came into the picture: Was God everywhere and invisible as he was told? Could his dead grandfather be everywhere and invisible since he was with God?

He then became preoccupied with food and eating. He drew a picture of a little boy who ate Cheerios. As he ate, his stomach grew bigger and bigger. It expanded so far that it burst, and pieces of stomach descended all over the room. He became concerned with germs: Food that he brought to the therapy session could carry germs. He "accidentally" dropped his apple and rolled it on the floor, picking up dirt, and he then bit into it. In his drawings, the germs entered the body and went to the stomach. The stomach changed into a fish tank, and many live things (fish) were wiggling around the body. Then, in further drawings, all sorts of "doo" (feces) in brown crayon poured out of the person's anus, completely covering the picture and the room.

The therapist and child worked together in the "Body Book," further clarifying and drawing the "mixed-up" ideas that Mark had. He thought that maybe the way a mommy became pregnant was by eating food and germs; the more she ate the bigger the baby became in her tummy, and the moving baby inside was like a fish. Slowly the therapist could draw other real pictures that clarified pregnancy for Mark.

Mark also wondered how a big baby could come out. Where was the baby hole? Did it emerge from the anus? The therapist explained that many boys had this scary idea. Again the therapist slowly drew and explained the anatomy of the mother, and how the child emerges, as he clarified Mark's ideas. He even kept a rubber band in the Body Book to explain the elasticity of the birth canal. His parents reported Mark's increasing periods of excitement followed by new periods of calm.

During one period of excitement, Mark became preoccupied with matches and had strong desires to get into bed with his brothers. In his sessions he became active and agitated. He no longer wanted to draw. He brought in a long nail or a pencil and colored the tips red. He gave the therapist these instruments and wanted him to touch his (Mark's) stomach (the instruments had fire on the tip). This was very exciting— the stomach would "burst." Mark wanted to be the passive, impregnated partner, and for a period he even sang "Here Comes the Bride" as he approached the office.

Again the therapist could control the exciting play (e.g., "Maybe we need to stop for a few minutes now, since this seems too exciting"). Mark was now bringing to the session his concept of intercourse (the frightening mommy bed and daddy bed noted earlier), which therapist and child could slowly discuss and draw at a pace that Mark could tolerate. The therapist could also discuss Mark's wish to be a woman. Mark sometimes had a very strong wish to be a mommy, to have babies inside and have a daddy touch him with a penis. The therapist told him that this was a wish that all boys had at times. (Mark had identified strongly with his powerful mother.) It was a very scary idea for him, because sometimes he wanted his "dick" to fall off so he could be just like a girl. Then he became very frightened, but this was just a fantasy idea. Working through Mark's passive wishes was a critical aspect of the therapeutic work, as his castration anxiety was very intense.

The therapeutic work at this period of time addressed a mixture of issues related to Mark's neurotic conflicts and developmental needs. Certainly a central conflict for Mark was his intense underlying wish to be a girl and his associated passive sexual wishes. He seemed to identify with his mother and expressed this in all of his pregnancy and baby-caring wishes. These wishes, however, were highly anxiety producing because of the castration wishes they promoted. A major factor in this youngster's overt driven hypermasculinity, defiance, and toughness was the need to deny and defend against the internal feminine drive. One of the major goals of treatment was to have these underlying impulses emerge, have the youngster accept some of these wishes inside himself (he was predominantly heterosexual), and help him understand that the fear of these internal feminine wishes drove him to prove inappropriately that he was the toughest boy in the neighborhood.

However, as therapist and child worked on these central issues, there emerged many other sexual fantasies that were a normal part of childhood. Mark explicated oral (food) fantasies of impregnation, anal fantasies of childbirth, a major denial of intercourse (daddies make babies in the hospital), and a denial of sexual differences (boys can have babies). Part of the natural task of childhood is struggling with all of these sexual theories and slowly accepting the reality of the "facts of life." It is clear that in this process the therapist had many opportunities to help Mark with these natural developmental sexual concepts as well as the central conflict that was causing him major problems. In some aspects of this work on sexual distortions, the work with Mark was ego-supportive (clarifying misconceptions). In work with children particularly, there is a need for an admixture of interpretation processes and ego-supportive elements (Kennedy & Moran, 1991). Thus, an important aspect of child psychotherapy is that the therapist comes to function as a "developmental facilitator" whereby he or she will clarify and interpret manifestations of development directly. Beiser, in a recent article (Beiser, 1995) discusses the special identifications the child makes with the therapist in intensive treatments.

COUNTERREACTIONS TO
THE CHILD PATIENT

It has been commonly recognized that there are unusual pressures and stresses in work with children (A. Freud, 1965; Bornstein, 1948; Chethik, 1969). These pressures produce strong internal reactions within the therapist. Some authors describe these internal reactions as countertransference reactions (countertransference, as it is often understood, refers to special feelings a child may elicit in a therapist that stem from the therapist's unique childhood experiences and his or her own latent neurotic tendencies). In work with children, however, there are many reactions that are dramatically evoked in all therapists by the very fact of having a child patient. These common reactions often make the course of treatment difficult and impede empathy and understanding of the small patient.

One of the major feelings a child therapist must endure in his work is *bewilderment* and *complete disorientation*. For example, in the early stages of the treatment with Mark there were sudden strong eruptions of aggression, excitement, panic, and incoherent disorder, and the therapist found himself confused and anxious. The child patient does not readily provide a context for his eruptive behavior. The therapist is flooded with questions. What does this eruptive material mean? What element is uppermost? What has caused the breakthrough? How shall it be handled? But often, with the acting-out child, the therapist has little time to think. At times he or she needs to act, although there may be much the therapist does not understand. In the first period of work with Mark, the therapist quickly moved to control the chaos—setting up rules, putting toys away, holding the child.

One of the affects child therapists need to come to terms with in dealing with the "acting out" that many child patients bring is the *anger* that is induced. It is important to appreciate the intensity of the response that 6-year-old Marks can produce. Winnicott (1965) noted that in child work "objective hate" can emerge and that such feelings often have an objective basis. This recognition is important in preventing the therapist from feeling a great deal of internal guilt, which can immobilize a therapist's capacity to work with the child. During Mark's eruptive and explosive periods, the therapist scheduled early morning appointments. The purpose was to get the chaotic hour out of the way so that he could have the rest of the day clear and relatively peaceful. It was certainly not unusual to anticipate the hour with Mark with a certain sense of dread.

The acting out produced by a child is not confined to the office alone. How the child uses the highly charged materials after the session ends is often a troubling question to the therapist. Because of the state of the child's ego, the demarcation between thought, wish, and fantasy, on the one hand, and action and behavior, on the other hand, is not always clear to the child. To what extent did Mark's "lion feelings" of the hour become expressed as the bully on the playground? Would the invulnerable "Mighty Mouse" emerging in Mark's sessions induce more daredevil exploits in the neighborhood? Child therapists often work with a certain anxiety about what the treatment may evoke in the child, as reality testing as an ego function is less well developed.

At times, in work with young children, the therapist is faced with a sense of *helplessness* because the child is dependent on his parents and family. When there are changes in the family (separation, divorce, illnesses, etc.) or ongoing influences that clearly affect the child, the therapist often experiences intense frustration as he or she clearly witnesses the changes in the child and the treatment process. Although Mark's mother, Mrs. L, slowly became amenable to undoing her strong need to reinforce and idealize Mark's "heroic" behavior, it was extremely difficult to witness this affirmation of his pathology in the early phases of the work with Mark. The therapist came to know that his efforts with Mark would be fruitless unless the mother became emotionally able to give up the gratification she received from her son's "manly" exploits.

In our work with children, recognizing the contribution parents make to the pathology in the child inevitably produces "*rescue fantasies*" within the therapist. The vulnerable little patient often evokes the wish to parent the child and protect the child from the negative influence of the "bad parent." These underlying impulses can undermine the treatment process. Will the therapist convey his or her indictment of the parents and disturb the alliance he or she has with them? Will the therapist inappropriately seek to "make up" for the parents' deprivation in his or her contacts with the child and thereby distort the therapist's therapeutic posture? These are some of the potential pitfalls induced by the rescue fantasy.

Although the state of the child's ego, his dependence, and his hesitant motivation do cause "wear and tear" on the therapist, there are also some unique pleasures the child therapist can experience.

For example, Mark, the stormy and trying 6-year-old, after a period of time, could begin to identify and discuss his out-of-control behavior. As noted earlier, he said during one session, "I have a lion inside me. And the wild lion gets me into a lot of trouble." One day, after a wretched hour, he commented with much sadness, "You know, it's just very hard for me to be good." Later in his treatment he discussed his terrifying dreams. He felt there was a little God inside him. This little God made bad dreams come at night when he was a bad boy during the day.

At times, in the treatment of the young child, we are involved in helping fundamental institutions necessary for growth emerge in the child. In Mark's statements one saw the beginning of new institutions. The "little God" inside him was the dawning awareness of his conscience and superego development. Seeing a lion inside himself, witnessing this wild part, indicated a beginning ego observer and self-evaluator. As thought and verbalization grew, as his affects could be put into words, Mark's destructive behavior came under control and new functions began to develop.

The therapist also recognizes that the child, by the very nature of being a child, has had a relatively short period of illness as compared with an adult. One does not have to undo a whole lifetime of entrenched and reinforced defenses or deal with an overlay of reality choices that have already been made on the basis of pathology. The changes in a child can be especially substantial and fundamental, and these changes can be the source of considerable gratification for the therapist.

The specific counterreactions identified earlier are not, in themselves, unique to the child practitioner. Bewilderment, anger, and helplessness are feelings that are part of everyone's practice. In addition to these internal negative feelings, the therapist often has positive affects (e.g., desires to protect the child against his helplessness) that can also form major roadblocks in the course of treatment. It is suggested that the intensity of these feelings is much stronger in work with children, that one experiences them much more frequently, and that these internal reactions come to form a very basic fact of the therapeutic work. It is important for the practitioner's own therapeutic self-esteem to distinguish these reactions from countertransference feelings. It is often reassuring, and perhaps essential, for the therapist to recognize within him- or herself the naturalness of these intense reactions in his or her work with children. In Brandell's book (1992) on countertransference he includes a number of chapters that discuss the internal reactions of therapists in specific situations that include racial and cultural differences, severely disturbed adolescents, eating disorders, borderline children, substance-abusing adolescents, and abused children.

BIBLIOGRAPHY

Ackerman, N. (1958). *Psychodynamics of Family Life*. New York: Basic Books.

Anthony, J. (1964). Communicating therapeutically with the child. *Journal of the American Academy of Child Psychiatry* 3:106–125.

Anthony, J. (1982). The comparable experiences of a child and adult analyst. *Psychoanalytic Study of the Child* 37:339–366.

Anthony, J. (1986). The contributions of child psychoanalysis to psychoanalysis. Psychoanalytic Study of the Child 41:61–88.

Bartholomew, K., & Horowitz, L. (1991). Attachment styles among young adults. *Journal of Personality and Social Psychology* 61:226–244.

Beiser, H. (1995). A follow-up of child analysis: The analyst as a real person. *The Psychoanalytic Study of the Child* 50:106–121.

Bornstein, B. (1948). Emotional barriers in the understanding and treatment of young children. *American Journal of Orthopsychiatry* 18:691–697.

Bowlby, J. (1988). *A Secure Base: Parent–Child Attachment and Healthy Human Development*. New York: Basic Books.

Brandell, J. (Ed.) (1992). *Countertransference in Psychotherapy with Children and Adolescents*. New Jersey/Northvale: Jason Aronson.

Chethik, M. (1969). The emotional "wear and tear" of child therapy. *Smith College Studies in Social Work* (Feb):147–156.

Chethik, M. (1976). Work with parents: Treatment of the parent–child relationship. *Journal of the American Academy of Child Psychiatry* 15:453–463.

Curtis, H. (1979). The concept of the therapeutic alliance. Implications for the "widening scope." *Journal of the American Psychoanalytic Association* 27(Suppl.):159–192.

Cutter, A., & Hallowitz, D. (1982). Different approaches to the treatment of the child and the parents. *American Journal of Orthoprychiatry* 22:152–159.

Davies, D. (1999). *Child Development: A Practitioner's Guide*. New York: Guilford Press.

Fraiberg, S. (1954). Counseling for parents of the very young child. *Social Casework* 35:47–57.

Freud, A. (1965). *Normality and Pathology in Childhood*. New York: International University Press.

Harley, M. (1986). Child analysis, 1947–1984: A retrospective. *Psychoanalytic Study of the Child* 41:129–154.

Kennedy, H., & Moran, G. (1991). Reflections on the aim of child analysis. *Psychoanalytic Study of the Child* 46:181–197.

Kessler, J. (1966). *Psychopathology of Childhood*. Englewood Cliffs, NJ: Prentice-Hall.

Kohrman, R., Fineberg, H., Gelman, R., & Weiss, S. (1971). Techniques of child analysis. *International journal of Psychoanalysis* 52:487–497.

Main, M., & Hesse, E. (1990). Parent's Unresolved Traumatic Experiences are related to Infant Disorganized Attachment Status. In M. T. Greenberg, D. Cicchetti, & E. M. Cummings (Eds.), *Attachment in Pre-School Years* (pp. 161–184). Chicago: University of Chicago Press.

Main, M., Kaplan, N., & Cassidy, J. (1985). Security in infancy, childhood, and adulthood. In I. Bretherton & E. Waters (Eds.), Growing points of attachment theory and research. *Monographs of the Society for Research in Child Development*, 50(1–2, Serial No. 209), 66–106.

Olden, C. (1953). On adult empathy with children. *Psychoanalytic Study of the Child* 8:lll–126.

Peller, L. (1954). Libidinal phases, ego development and play. *The Psychoanalytic Study of the Child* 9:178–198.

Rees, K. (1978). The child's understanding of his past. Cognitive factors in reconstruction with children. *Psychoanalytic Study of the Child* 33:237–259.

Ritvo, S. (1978). The psychoanalytic process in childhood. *Psychoanalytic Study of the Child* 33:295–305.

Sandler, J., Kennedy, H., & Tyson, P. (1980). *The Techniques of Child Analysis: Discussions with Anna Freud*. Cambridge, MA: Harvard University Press.

Tyson, R., & Tyson, P. (1986). The concept of transference in child psychoanalysis. *Journal of the American Academy of Child Psychiatry* 25:30–39.

Winnicott, D. W. (1965). *The Maturational Process and the Facilitating Environment*. New York: International Universities Press.

2

∼

The Process of Assessment
and Its Role
in the Treatment Process

The purpose of this chapter is not merely to focus on the diagnostic process itself but also to illustrate how extensively a good assessment can orient the therapist to the specifics of an anticipated treatment. Initially, in this chapter, a full evaluation of a 6-year-old youngster is presented. A psychodynamic technical assessment of the case is then described, with specific treatment recommendations. This is followed by a discussion of how various aspects of the case may emerge and present themselves in the course of treatment. Although it is clear that no one can make absolute predictions about how a case will unfold or what new significant factors will become evident, the diagnostic context is an absolutely crucial one. The diagnostic backdrop is critical as the therapist seeks to make sense of and organize the unfolding material of the treatment hour. Therefore, this chapter is intended to serve as an example of the interweaving, the back-and-forth process of assessment and treatment.

THE EVALUATION PROCESS
OF EMANUEL R AND FAMILY

The evaluation consisted of two interviews with the mother, two sessions with Emanuel, one with the father, and reports from the pediatrician, nursery school, and first grade teacher. Emanuel was 6 years of age at the time of the evaluation, and his parents had been divorced for more than 2 years. Emanuel was the youngest in a sibship of three—two older sisters (Dorothy, age 11, and Cynthia, age 9) made up the rest of the family. All lived in a single home in an upper-middle-class community with the mother, while the father lived nearby in a smaller home to which the children had easy access and visited frequently.

The Initial Phone Call

In an initial phone call, Mrs. R said that she wished to have her son, Emanuel, evaluated. She indicated she had been worried about him for a long time. She said she was divorced, had contacted Emanuel's father, and that he was supportive of the evaluation and would participate. She asked about the fee. The therapist told her the fee he charged, and the mother indicated that the figure was acceptable to her. The therapist then provided directions to his office and set up a meeting with the mother.

The function of the initial session is partially a screening session to determine whether a full evaluation should occur. Parents usually describe the behavior problems and/or symptoms in the first session, and the chronicity or transitory nature of the difficulties. There are times when a parent is actually seeking treatment for him- or herself, or there may be a current crisis with a child that does not necessitate a full evaluation. When a determination is made, the therapist can then outline the process that will occur.

The therapist typically meets with the parent or parents (if an intact family) alone in that first meeting. Again, this is to determine whether a full evaluation should occur. In addition, the therapist can help the parents prepare the child for the evaluation should they decide to proceed.

First Interview: Mrs. R

Mrs. R was an attractive woman in her mid-30s who was markedly upset by rather chronic problems with her 6-year-old son. She felt that since the divorce (final separation occurred when Emanuel was 3½ years of age), her daughters had done extremely well in their development, but this was not true of her son. She was now completing her own undergraduate education and would shortly be looking for employment.

In the first interview the therapist asked the mother to describe the chronic problems she mentioned. She expressed great concern about the fighting relationship she had with Emanuel. She found she was furious with him almost all the time, and he fought back. He often would not accept her authority—for example, about eating or dressing. He was very stubborn and ended up saying, "I won't." Because she was bigger, his mother noted, she would win by subduing him with force, but they often ended up screaming and yelling, with Mrs. R spanking her child. She hated what she thought she had descended to. Emanuel also embarrassed her a great deal. He had temper tantrums with the children of her friends, and he was extremely bossy and controlling of all friends. She hated to hear his voice telling others what to do. In all of this descriptive material, the therapist asked for specific examples. The mother felt that Emanuel also stood in the way of her relationships with men. Because he could be so impossible and made a fuss when she was going out, she felt impeded in her ability to become seriously involved with a man. Who would want her with this little hellion attached?

In response to the therapist's questions, she related that the incident that made her decide to call for an evaluation had occurred over the recent Christmas vacation. Emanuel was very angry and suddenly said directly that he wanted to stab his mother with a knife. To verbalize these things actually made him calm down, and they had a very good time for several days. She had ambivalent feelings about this incident—she was scared about how angry he was, but she also wondered whether the situation would improve if he could express a lot of his feelings in therapy.

The therapist asked whether there were other things that worried her about her son. Mrs. R noted that Emanuel had been a bed wetter throughout his life (almost every night), and although he was bright, his teachers thought he was not working up to his academic potential.

At this point the therapist felt that a full evaluation should occur, because there were indeed long-standing difficulties, apprised the mother of his assessment, and outlined the process. He needed several sessions with the mother to learn about Emanuel's developmental history, her own history, and the marriage with her former husband. He explained that how a person was raised as a child often shapes how he or she is as a parent. He would also meet with Emanuel several times, and because there were some school difficulties, he would need to contact both public and nursery school teachers, if possible. He suggested that the father call him for an appointment. After he gathered this material, he would integrate it and share his impressions and recommendations with her, Emanuel, and the father.

For most of the rest of the session, Mrs. R discussed her marriage and the difficulties she and her husband had had. They had never had a good marriage, and part of the difficulty lay with her. She admired her husband, but she had never loved him. He was an outstanding business executive, friendly, warm, and successful, but they had never felt close to each other. They could not talk with each other, and, frankly, the more competent her husband was, the less adequate she felt as a person. She believed that there was greater distance between them after Emanuel was born, despite the fact that they had hoped another child would bring them together. Mr. R had always been nice and polite and had been even more effective with the handling of Emanuel during his infancy and early years than she herself. Truthfully, at times, she had felt he was showing her up.

At the end of the session, she wondered whether she could ever be a competent mother at all to a son—maybe Emanuel would be better off with his father. Tears flooded her eyes when she said that maybe this evaluation should consider where custody should reside.

Second Interview: Mrs. R

In the second interview, Mrs. R spontaneously said she was very upset about the session of last week. She had felt dizzy as she left and nauseous as she had entered her car. Could she really give up Emanuel? She found that idea very difficult, and she felt very sad. She loved him and said she wanted to rear him unless the therapist found some very compelling and clear reason that they should not live together.

In terms of further history, Mrs. R noted that she had wanted another baby more than anything in the world, and she was the most happy in her life during her pregnancies. She was, however, a perfectionist. She had taken Lamaze lessons, as she had before, and had not really expected the delivery to hurt her. She had been so surprised by the pain and depressed by her inability to bear it that she was initially angry with Emanuel. But it was a good first year—she had enjoyed feeding and holding him, buying his clothes, bunting, and other items, and recalled that she had loved to look at him peacefully lying in his crib.

Emanuel was a very active toddler and hard to keep up with. By then her marriage was deteriorating, and she knew she was often angry and depressed and very impatient with Emanuel. As he neared 2 years of age she began toilet training him, and he was quickly successful. But after a few weeks he totally refused the potty, and she could not cajole him. Her use of force, however, also did not work. He soiled then for more than a year, and finally, when he was 3½ and she made him wash out his pants, the soiling problem disappeared forever. She has always had problems, however, with getting Emanuel to put away his toys, papers, and other things. It is quite clear which rooms of her house Emanuel has recently been in—the disorder is very evident.

The therapist asked about Mrs. R's current living situation. Mrs. R talked openly about her boyfriend, Larry, who had been living in the home for the past year. She was upset that Emanuel made believe that Larry did not exist and hardly spoke to him. Larry was a "natural" with children, but he felt that Emanuel was a terribly spoiled youngster. In terms of her relationship with Larry, Mrs. R believed that he wanted to marry her, but she was terribly unsure. She was physically attracted to Larry but felt unable to really talk with him about any feelings or sensitive matters. They maintained the current arrangement partly because she hated to be lonely, but she was not sure the relationship was going anywhere.

Mrs. R spoke of her own history. She recalled a very unhappy childhood. Her parents had separated and divorced when she was 18 but fought all the time during her early years. No one seemed to care about her—her parents were preoccupied with themselves, and she recalled "disappearing into the woodwork" so no one would notice her. Her mother told her she was an "accident," and her father's concern had been that she marry so that she would not be a financial burden on him. She also recalled being very competitive with her brothers, who were 2 and 4 years older than she. Mrs. R thoughtfully speculated that her feelings of inadequacy as a child had been a central problem in her marriage. She had felt so small in contrast to her husband that she could not stand it—this was an important awareness derived from her own treatment, which she began when her marriage became precarious. Her treatment had lasted for several years through her subsequent divorce.

At the end of the session, Mrs. R described again several incidents with Emanuel that troubled her greatly. For example, with good intentions and a determination to have a good time, she had taken Emanuel for an afternoon to the science museum. He had taken over and had tried to determine what exhibits they would see, how long she should spend looking at fossils, and so on. By the end of the trip she had been furious. The power struggle seemed ever present.

In achieving a meaningful history of a child, the facts of a developmental history are not enough. It is the task of the evaluator to attempt to construct in his or her mind the emotional climate in which the child patient grew up. Thus, there is a need to understand the emotional life of the parents as much as possible. Having parents describe the family atmosphere and events during the years of the child's life and learning of the childhood history of the parents themselves helps the therapist to understand the quality of parental functioning. Mrs. R highlighted the struggle between the parents during Emanuel's early years. In other cases, financial constraints, absorption in professional development, moves, or deaths of significant relatives can be important in understanding families, because these events can significantly encroach on an adult's available energy to parent effectively.

Emanuel R: First Interview

Emanuel was a robust, pleasant looking youngster. He initially looked apprehensive about meeting the therapist. Because he wore a baseball cap, the therapist asked him about his interest in the Detroit Tigers. Emanuel, however, went quickly for the toys in the room, as they seemed safe and familiar. He took out all sorts of toys—trucks, soldiers, cowboys—and a chaotic mess seemed to ensue. Soldiers were killing monsters who were killing trucks who were killing other soldiers. The therapist asked questions about the fighting (Who was fighting? Why? etc.) There appeared to be no story line, and the violence, which was very evident, seemed to have little form. As the play went on, the therapist felt there was some evidence of anxiety: questions regarding the details of the story met with little or no comment. Emanuel, however, seemed to attend when the therapist spoke about why he was coming for sessions. The therapist noted that his mommy felt that Emanuel was unhappy, and that this unhappiness came from worries. His mom felt he showed this by being angry a lot, wetting the bed, and having trouble having friends. The therapist was now trying to figure out Emanuel's worries by seeing him, his mom, and his dad. After he had seen them a few times, he would think about Emanuel's worries and give Emanuel his ideas about them and how these ideas might help Emanuel.

Emanuel picked up on the therapist's comment about "worries" and said he had bad dreams. He was scared when he went to sleep and sometimes stayed under the covers. He was visited in his dreams by monsters from the dead—from the underground. They sprayed in people's faces, and this killed them. He had a dream in which a monster came upon a family that was eating dinner, and it sprayed into the daddy's face. Emanuel shifted from the dream and immediately began talking about his mother's boyfriend, Larry, whom he said he liked very much. Larry worked a lot on his house and fixed things, and Emanuel liked to help him. Maybe, he said, his mom and Larry would get married in the summer.

It is interesting to follow the progression of Emanuel's thoughts. His "good feelings" about Larry emerged immediately after a dream about his daddy being killed. This was a reaction formation that was noted by the therapist but not commented on directly. This kind of material would be used to understand Emanuel's conflicts (discussed later in the chapter) but would have been premature to raise with the child at this point.

Emanuel R: Second Interview

The therapist began the second session by noting that he and Emanuel were still finding out about his worries. Sometimes drawings and stories about the drawings helped to explain inside worries. Emanuel began by telling about other bad dreams. He had dreamt that his mother was a witch, and in some dreams she had been holding a dead body. He became anxious by this revelation, and he ran to check on his mother in the waiting room.

Emanuel worked on several drawings, and he told a story as he drew. A boy and his mother went to sleep together in the bedroom. When the boy was asleep the mother turned into a witch. She cast a magical spell on herself to kill herself. She did this by eating a poison apple. Bats then flew around and ate her body. The boy awakened and saw this skeleton, and it began to chase him. He was very scared and ran away and went to live with his daddy.

The therapist noted that sometimes Emanuel seemed to get very angry with his mom. He agreed he was angry with Larry and his mom. When he went to sleep, he said, they left him and he was alone. Many times, they went walking together and did not want him there! They talked all the time, and he did not know what they were talking about. Because they only talked to themselves, he was going to get even. He would not even talk to them or listen to his mother when she told him to do something. Emanuel expressed his anger with a good deal of affect.

At the end of the session the therapist noted that boys can get very, very angry with their mommies. Later they often feel bad, because they need them and also want things to go well. Maybe the therapist could help him and his mom get along better and be happier, if the therapist knew more about the angry feelings he and his mom had.

In the early stages of an evaluation or treatment, it is helpful to give a child some glimpse of how therapy may be helpful. Emanuel was very angry with his mother but also clearly pained by the problems between them. The therapist took this opportunity to make this a conscious issue and indicated that it was an important one, which he would attempt to help Emanuel and his mother resolve. The purpose of such early comments is to foster investment in this new, strange process.

School Report: First Grade Teacher

Generally, Emanuel's teacher believed that she had learned to handle him and that he had "settled down" since the start of the year. She had learned to be very firm with him, and his desk was near hers. Since she had provided this "structure," his learning and behavior had improved, although he was having significant difficulty with his reading progress. He was potentially one of the smartest children she had seen in a long time. His vocabulary, insight, general knowledge, and reasoning attested to his capabilities, but she thought that he seemed to have "a lot of turmoil going on inside of him." Earlier, Emanuel had chosen to associate with a large, very aggressive youngster who was the class problem, but more recently kept away from him.

Nursery School

Emanuel had attended nursery school and kindergarten in this program. Overall, Emanuel was not a major "acter-outer," but he tended to associate with the more difficult children; for a period of time, he loved the use of "bad" and "bathroom" language. He did very well with firm teachers and had difficulties with lax teachers.

He had some inhibitions academically, but during the latter half of his kindergarten year, he flourished in math and science, although he had some problems in reading preparation skills.

Interview with Mr. R

Mr. R was a successful, handsome business executive in his mid-30s who enjoyed his profession. The requirements of his job demanded that he travel a good deal, and he liked moving about. He had never remarried, although he had had a number of relationships since his divorce.

He visited with Emanuel and his sisters twice weekly (usually for a good part of the weekend) except when he was out of town. He had supported his ex-wife and family financially and was willing to support and pay for treatment. He was aware of Emanuel's difficulties with his mother, but he had not observed these directly. Emanuel was never a problem with his father. He was very well behaved, and they thoroughly enjoyed each other's company. He knew that the division of labor in raising Emanuel had not been totally fair, and he tried to take the children for weekends so that his ex-wife could have time for special things she wanted to do.

He had some concern about Emanuel's sexual interests. Mr. R at times had had women friends over when Emanuel visited. Recently Emanuel had acted very seductively with these women, and Mr. R was uncomfortable with the precocious quality of his remarks and gestures. He expressed a desire to explore this actively in parent guidance sessions in the future.

PSYCHODYNAMIC TECHNICAL ASSESSMENT

Tbe major topics to be addressed in a technical assessment are included in the following outline. An illustration of such an assessment is presented, using the case material of Emanuel and his family.

I. Drive Assessment (libidinal and aggressive)
   Include psychosexual phase development, phase level, and quality object relations (mostly in regard to libido), quantity, and distribution with regard to aggression
II. Ego Assessment
   A. Defensive functions—preferred defenses, appropriateness, and efficiency
   B. Quality of object relations—extent of capacity to relate
   C. Relation to reality—capacity to adapt
   D. Nature of thinking processes—abstract versus concrete, utilization of fantasy
   E. Drive regulation and control—development of drive endowment, superego function; assessing degree of impulsivity, frustration tolerance, and attention span
   F. Autonomous functions—intelligence, memory (immediate and remote, lapses or distortions), motor function

(coordination and use of body language), perception
(distortions—organic or psychologic), and language
  G. Synthetic function—assessing capacity to integrate and
     organize experience
  H. Assessment of ego's general functioning in light of the
     preceding items, relative to age and developmental stage
III. Superego Assessment
     Broadly assess nature and extent of guilt versus fear of ex-
     ternal authority
IV. Genetic–Dynamic Formulation of Child
     Discuss major sources of conflict related to:
       psychosexual phase of development
       external and internal conflicts relative to child
       major identifications and their contributions to child's
       adaptations
 V. Treatment Recommendations

This outline, by itself, will not give the reader enough information to proceed with a diagnostic assessment. It is necessary to be
more familiar with the drives and the attendant phases of development, with the ego and the specific defenses, with how the superego
works and manifests itself. To discuss all these issues is beyond the
scope of this book, and the reader is referred to several important
sources that will explicate these issues. See A. Freud (1965) and
Tyson & Tyson (1990). The creator of this technical assessment is
Anna Freud, through her work at the Hampstead Clinic. General reviews of her assessment contributions are also discussed by a number
of authors (Mayes & Cohen, 1996; Yorke, 1996). For a further up-
date of this profile, the reader is referred to Greenspan, Hattesberg,
& Cullander (1991) and their discussion on assessment.
    The purpose of the assessment is to shed light on specific prob-
lematic areas and explicate the underlying forces that have created
the difficulties. Emanuel presented several issues. (1) The major manifest difficulty was the fighting relationship with his mother, but the
problems seemed to spread into other areas of their relationship as
well, and to a limited degree affected Emanuel's relationship with
other authorities. He was ready to fight rules, evidenced messy
behavior generally, and had temper tantrums. Emanuel's "bossy"
behavior was also evident with peers. (2) In addition, he had been
enuretic at night for a number of years, and the bed-wetting pattern

seemed related to internal conflicts (e.g., often after nightmares or bad dreams, the wetting occurred). (3) Emanuel seemed to evidence some problems at school—although he was bright, he did not work up to his potential, and he had particular difficulty with learning to read. How would we explain these symptoms and behavior problems?

As an approach to making the assessment, the outline is designed in a particular way. Sections I, II, and III focus on three major institutions of the mind (the id, ego, and superego), and these should be examined separately. Section IV (genetic dynamic formulation) is conceived as an attempt to integrate the first three sections and to describe the child's internal struggles (dynamic formulation) and trace the factors in his history that influenced these struggles (genetic formulation). After one has made this formulation, a diagnosis of the child would be more evident, and the course of treatment can be clearer.

Application of the Outline

I. Drive Assessment

There was a good deal of evidence that Emanuel had reached the phallic and oedipal levels of development. This was suggested by the dream of going into the bedroom with his mother and wishes to sleep with her. Emanuel's relationships were "triangulated," which is typical of children in the oedipal phase of development. He saw Larry, his mother's boyfriend, as an intense rival, and he was jealous of their activities and the time they spent together. Emanuel's sexual interests were also expressed in his seductive behavior with his father's girlfriends.

Emanuel was having major difficulty dealing with this phase of development. His phallic sexuality seemed very destructive to him. The sprayer (penis symbol in the dream described in the first hour) killed the daddy when it was squirted into his face. Emanuel expressed fear of destruction as he experienced rivalry with Daddy and Larry. Intercourse was very frightening to him. After he and his mother retired to the bedroom, his mother turns into a witch and skeletons chase him. These frightening and bad dreams that Emanuel described suggested that he feared punishment for his destructive competitive strivings and his sexual wishes.

There were also problems stemming from the anal phase of development. Some of his sexuality seemed to be expressed in anal terms. The material suggested that some of his power struggles with his mother were exciting and had aspects of sadomasochistic interplay.

Emanuel clearly had difficulty with his aggressive drives as well. He had trouble controlling his aggression, particularly with his mother. Some of his difficulties related to the phallic rivalry described earlier. He also evidenced difficulties stemming from the anal phase, which he expressed in temper tantrums, messiness, and controlling behavior.

II. Ego Assessment

Basically, Emanuel seemed well endowed, and all of his ego functions seemed intact and well developed (intelligence, perception, memory, etc.). In terms of object development, he certainly had reached object constancy (basic capacity for a stable libidinal attachment to people), although there were some problems in the resolution of ambivalence. Emanuel tended to idealize his father and devalue his mother.

Emanuel made use of several prominent defenses. When he was frightened of the aggression of others, he utilized the mechanism of *identification with the aggressor* (e.g., when he felt his mother would attack, he became the attacker). Emanuel had considerable problems with his aggression, and he commonly engaged in *projection*, ascribing the forbidden feelings to others around him. Another major defensive maneuver was *regression*. Emanuel seemed to be frightened of sexual and loving oedipal feelings, and he moved from these affects (e.g., toward his mother) to earlier, preoedipal forms of relationship.

At times Emanuel appeared impulsive when aggressive breakthroughs seemed to emerge. This reaction served several purposes for him. Sometimes his ego seemed to have difficulty regulating his drives, and he was overwhelmed by the strength of his feelings. In addition, the choice of his defense (identification with the aggressor) permitted the open expression and discharge of his aggression.

III. Superego Assessment

Emanuel did not have a fully internalized superego, and he depended somewhat on authorities (mother and teachers) for controls. He had a growing sense of right and wrong but imagined that many sanctions would be unduly harsh (stemming, in part, from the projection of his aggression). Because of the problems he had with aggression, he anticipated (imagined) cruel and destructive punishments for his transgressions.

IV. Genetic–Dynamic Formulation

Emanuel was a youngster struggling to reach the oedipal phase of development, but conflicts at this stage became very problematic for him. He was quite frightened that his phallic behavior (both sexual and aggressive) was very destructive to others and that expressing these phase-appropriate feelings would have terrible consequences for him. Sprayers (penises) killed daddies, and sleeping with mother (bedroom fantasy) was associated with terrifying witches and skeletons. He was frightened that his urges were too destructive and powerful. Emanuel tended to retreat to many forms of anal functioning, where he felt safer. For example, rather than expressing the sexuality and love feelings of the oedipal phase, he maintained a fighting, controlling (anal) relationship with his mother.

Stemming from the history, there appeared to be three major factors that contributed to Emanuel's feelings that his phallic and oedipal strivings were destructive:

1. During Emanuel's anal phase of development he struggled with his mother around issues of autonomy (toilet training history) and as a consequence built up a reservoir of anger in relation to his sexual and aggressive affects, which he carried further into his development. Affects of rage, negativism, and defiance were legacies of unresolved problems of the anal phase.

2. In addition, his fears of power were markedly exacerbated by his parents' separation and divorce during his oedipal years. In his fantasy, he was an "oedipal victor" who had gotten rid of his father, expressed by the dream in which the monster kills the daddy with his spray. The separation had actually occurred when Emanuel was 3½ years old. Fathers, at this point in development, normally serve as a natural inhibitor for the aggressive/sexual fantasies of little boys. This loss appeared to have reinforced Emanuel's sense of omnipotence, as little boys have a common wish to expel their fathers from the family. This event contributed to the fear of his destructive power. The absence of the father also appeared to have exacerbated the problematic interactions between mother and son, inasmuch as

the father was not there to serve as a buffer in this primary relationship. These two factors became problems internalized within Emanuel.

3. The third factor and barrier to oedipal resolution was an external factor, Mrs. R's feelings about Emanuel's masculine strivings. Mrs. R was clearly conflicted about her own relationships with men. She felt she was small and inadequate in comparison to the phallic strength of her husband (and probably, earlier, her father). She had competed unsuccessfully with her brothers. It appeared that Mrs. R saw her son's activity (both autonomy and phallic strivings) as destructive and also demeaning to her. Thus, on a day-to-day current basis, Mrs. R's sanctions made Emanuel's oedipal strivings difficult to express.

V. Treatment Recommendations

Twice-weekly, insight-oriented psychotherapy for Emanuel was recommended to help him to deal with his internalized conflicts. In making this recommendation, it was important to assess Emanuel's potential strengths for the task. Emanuel appeared to be an intelligent youngster who showed no problems in memory, perception, or motor or language functions. He related well in the two evaluative sessions, and he responded to the ideas of the therapist with dreams, drawings, and stories. His thinking processes and his ability to imagine and fantasize were intact. Despite the disturbance evident with his mother, Emanuel was able to function elsewhere with firm limits so that part of the problematic behavior was limited to his relationship with his mother. It was also clear that this was not a youngster who had given up. Emanuel struggled to reenter the phallic arena, and this was very apparent in his visits with his father.

Weekly parent guidance was recommended for the mother. A major task would be to help her to accept the phallic and masculine strivings in her youngster. Given the mother's history and general struggle with her own identity, this might not be easy. However, she had already had some therapy, and perhaps the insights gained could be used in relation to her son. She was also strongly motivated to help her son and could potentially feel enhanced by being an effective parent.

Intermittent parent guidance for the father was recommended. The purpose of this would be to support his investment and attachment to his son.

Summary

In summary, there were now a number of hypotheses gathered to explain Emanuel's presenting problems. The most complex issue was his aggressive behavior (outbursts with his mother, with Larry, and with other authorities). At times, Emanuel's behavior appeared to be a direct response to his mother's attacks or belittling behavior directed at her son. Emanuel's anger also seemed to be a direct expression of reactions to the "past" mother (of the anal toilet training period). Emanuel's fighting behavior was also defensive, as his belligerence was a more acceptable form of relating to his mother than the expression of the tenderness or sexuality of the oedipal period. In relation to men, Emanuel's angry behavior appeared to be the expression of his rivalry with an oedipal antagonist.

Similar oedipal themes seemed to explain his bed-wetting. At times, the symptom appeared to reflect the expression of phallic impulses in his dreams. Emanuel used his powerful "sprayer" to annihilate men. Bed-wetting also reflected his anxiety in punishment dreams. Does his penis become broken (the bed-wetting act) as an expression of his castration anxiety? The evaluation also suggested that because Emanuel struggled with fears regarding the expression of his power, some of his conflict may have been displaced to his intellectual power. It appeared that Emanuel needed to restrict his performance in school (associated with phallic performance), where he was expected to be competitive and rivalrous with others.

Diagnostically, using the conflict model (conflict between id, ego, and superego) described earlier, we can depict Emanuel's conflicts as shown in Table 2.1.

TABLE 2.1. Emmanuel's Structural Conflicts

Drive	→ Anxiety reaction	→ Ego response (response)	→ Behavior/ symptoms
I. Aggression Anal (sadism)	→ Fear of annihilation	→ Identification with the aggressor	→ Rage, temper, outbursts, messiness, etc.
Oedipal (competition)	→ Castration anxiety	→ Inhibition	→ School restriction
II. Libido Oedipal	→ Guilt/castration anxiety	→ Regression (in object relations)	→ Fighting interplay with mother

TREATMENT IMPLICATIONS

Although it is taken for granted that a diagnostic assessment has many implications for the treatment of a child, it is often not specifically articulated how the assessment can be used. The most obvious area is the setting of *treatment goals*. In most situations (as with Emanuel), symptoms and/or behavior problems develop because of unacceptable internal impulses. Insight into one's internal life can substantially modify how one reacts to these "negative" or forbidden parts of the self. Therefore, the diagnostic process can specify what aspects of the instinctual life seem to be most troubling. A goal would be to have the forbidden impulses expressed, discussed, and reintegrated via treatment into the child's psychic life.

In addition, part of the diagnostic appraisal focuses on the ego—the special responses the patient uses to ward off, repress, and defend against the conscious emergence of unacceptable impulses. These ego responses (e.g., defenses) are the typical forms the child patient uses to take flight from these troublesome aspects of the self. These responses will emerge in the treatment hour and become the specific forms of *resistance* the child will use in treatment. The diagnostic appraisal can therefore anticipate the specific resistances that may emerge.

Another area of anticipation is the nature of the *transferences* that will emerge in the course of therapy. (Both the concepts of "resistance" and "transference" in child work are more fully elaborated the Introduction to Part III.) Whom will the therapist come to represent as the result of problematic object relations of the past? What major past (or present) situations will be played out in the treatment hour? Understanding, through the diagnostic appraisal, the significant relationships during each phase of development, and the significant past events in a child's life, will allow the therapist to verbalize and reconstruct them as they emerge. The therapist can anticipate his transference role and the context in which it occurs.

These subjects are described in greater detail in the following sections.

Treatment Goals

What can we anticipate in the case of Emanuel? In terms of treatment goals, it is apparent that aspects of his rage and aggression are unacceptable to him and cause loss of self-esteem as well as negative reactions from people in his environment. In the course of treatment, we can anticipate that a fighting, rageful representation of Emanuel will emerge—perhaps directly with the therapist or in representational form through play. A major goal would be to help Emanuel put these affects (e.g., expressed in action, in play) into words and link them to real situations in his life. For example, Emanuel may be helped to say, "I hate my mother for such and such" as this emotion emerges in derivative play. With children, the process of verbalization modulates the raw affective drive components and helps a child order his instinctual life.

Further, Emanuel uses some "unacceptable" ways of expressing his anger. He can be enormously messy, and these aspects of his aggressive drive will emerge during the treatment hour. One could expect that at some point he will make a mess of the toys or some area of the treatment room. This would provide the opportunity for identifying Emanuel's "messy, angry feelings." A goal of the treatment may be to explicate this aspect of Emanuel's behaviors and slowly give him an understanding of how he developed them (for example, how boys love to be dirty when they are little, and if there are problems at that point, these feelings remain). The purpose of this kind of reconstruction of the aggressive drive would be to give his behavior some meaningful context and historical framework. This treatment insight can be helpful in beginning to modulate the harsh internal superego reactions (I am a terrible messy boy) to these impulses.

If the fighting play in the treatment hour (e.g., between a boy doll and a mommy doll) appears to be defending against oedipal issues, the therapeutic goal would be to illuminate the issues. The therapist can speak to Emanuel's fears of his tender or loving feelings toward his mother that cause him to fight with her. Again, the purpose would be to permit the expression of "forbidden" instinctual wishes so that Emanuel could move toward appropriate phase development.

This recognition of the nature of these conflicts as they emerge in the treatment hour can be enhanced enormously by an ordered diagnostic workup.

Resistance

What kind of resistances can we anticipate in the treatment hour with Emanuel? The diagnostic assessment highlights a number of typical defenses (e.g., identification with the aggressor, projection) that Emanuel utilizes, and one can expect that these forms of defense (resistance) will naturally emerge in interactions with the therapist.

For example, at some point in the course of the work, Emanuel will probably "act tough" and behave defiantly. Perhaps he will refuse to help to clean up at the end of the hour and instead dump the toys in defiance. He might throw clay pellets in the therapist's direction. The process of "identification with the aggressor" would then become apparent. With an understanding of the nature of the resistance, the therapist could interpret that "Emanuel becomes a tough guy when he imagines that the therapist will *force* him to clean up." This form of ego analysis can help Emanuel slowly become aware of his typical reactions to normal rules and expectations.

A similar process can be anticipated in relation to Emanuel's common use of projection. In the course of the work, Emanuel might become fearful of coming to his sessions. He could attribute all sorts of rage reactions to the therapist. The therapist, alerted to the defense/resistance mechanisms of projection, would have an opportunity to intervene and explain thus: "When Emanuel becomes angry, at times he pushes those feelings outside and onto the therapist. Now he has become scared of these angry feelings and scared the therapist will hurt him." The therapist could also draw parallels in Emanuel's life, to situations where this has happened on the playground, at home, or in other circumstances. If the typical defenses are anticipated, the therapist will be able to describe the distorted reactions as they emerge in the course of treatment and help the patient become aware of a major part of his personality—his ego functions.

Transference

All patients live out their feelings and experiences in the course of treatment rather than remember them. The history of the patient provides an important road map in helping the therapist locate the source of current unfolding action. What would Emanuel tend to reexperience?

One could anticipate that Emanuel would become provocative, messy, defiant, and bossy in his relationship with the therapist. Although this would include the process of "identification with the aggressor described earlier, in a larger context Emanuel would be recreating the maternal transference. He would be living out, with the therapist, some aspects of the sadomasochistic interplay he established with his mother during his early years. The therapist would become, for Emanuel, the controlling, dominating authority who would rob him of his products and freedom. This awareness would provide the therapist with an opportunity to identify the interplay verbally, reconstruct the past slowly, and help the patient see how he tends to replay these patterns inappropriately in critical areas of his current life. (The process of dealing with transference, reconstruction, and working through is elaborated in a number of cases in Part III.)

One can also anticipate another major form of transference based on Emanuel's past. Emanuel will probably be reactive during separations. Will he be concerned that the therapist may die in a plane crash when he goes on vacation? Will he worry that the therapist may never return? These separations would touch on feelings Emanuel had experienced when he "lost" his father at age 3½. One might comment to Emanuel that when he worries that the therapist will never come back, these feelings resemble those he might have had as a little boy when his dad and mommy split up. Often in divorced families, little children feel they were the ones who really made their daddies go away. Such a transference experience can provide opportunities to explore the impact and vicissitudes of his special father loss during the early phases of Emanuel's oedipal period.

There are clearly many other possible forms of resistance, transference, or reconstruction that one can anticipate in reviewing Emanuel's assessment. In the course of work with the child patient, the current material will slowly acquire specific meanings as one reassesses it in the context of the child's history and metapsychology. It is the diagnostic framework, then, the history and dynamic formulations, that make the ongoing material of the treatment hour intelligible.

BIBLIOGRAPHY

Freud, A. (1965). *Normality and Pathology in Childhood*. New York: International Universities Press.

Greenspan, S. (1982). *The Clinical Interview of the Child*. New York: McGraw-Hill.

Greenspan, S., Hattesberg, J., & Cullander, C. (1991). A developmental approach to systematic personality assessment. In S. Greenspan & G. Pollock (Eds.), *The Course of Life, Vol. III*. Madison, CT: IUP.

Group for the Advancement of Psychiatry. (1957). *The Diagnostic Process in Child Psychiatry*. Report No. 38. New York: Group for the Advancement of Psychiatry.

Mayes, C., & Cohen, D. (19960. Anna Freud and developmental psychoanalytic psychology. *Psychoanalytic Study of the Child* 51:117–141.

McDonald, M. (1965). The psychiatric evaluation of children. *Journal of the American Academy of Child Psychiatry* 4:569–612.

Nagera, H. (1963). The developmental profile: Notes on some practical considerations regarding its use. *Psychoanalytic Study of the Child* 18:511–540.

Newbauer, P. (1963). Psychoanalytic contributions to the nosology of childhood psychic disorders. *Journal of the American Psychoanalytic Association* 11:595–604.

Sandler, J., & Freud, A. (1965). *The Analysis of Defense*. New York: International Universities Press.

Sandler, J., Kennedy, H., & Tyson, R. (1980). *The Technique of Child Psychoanalysis: Discussions with Anna Freud*. Cambridge, MA: Harvard University Press.

Tyson, P., & Tyson, R. (1990). *Psychoanalytic Theories of Development: An Integration*. New Haven, CT: Yale University Press.

Yorke, C. (1996). Diagnosis in clinical practice. *Psychoanalytic Study of the Child* 51:190–214.

3

∽

The Central Role of Play

Chapter 1 presented some initial discussion of the child's need for action and the function of play. It is difficult to function as a child therapist without understanding the extraordinary role of *play*—not only
in a child's life and in the process of child therapy, but also in development and effective functioning in adulthood as well. Shengold, in a
symposium on the "Meaning of Play" (Shengold, 1988) noted that
there should be new criteria for good mental health. He proclaimed
that in addition to Freud's enumeration of *work* and *love*, we should
add the capacity to *play*. Plaut (1979) introduced this idea: "From a
psychological point of view, love, work and play are three ideal types
of action."

PLAY DEFINED

What is the special power of play? The basic assumption we have in
psychodynamic theory is that problems, anxieties, and symptoms
emerge because of conflict—conflict between drives on the one hand,
and the ego and superego on the other. For example, a 5-year-old girl
may feel that her rage (the aggressive drive) toward a new male sibling is totally unacceptable (to her ego and superego), and she can
maladaptively inhibit much of her aggressive functioning to ward off
internal self-reproach. Typically, these developmental impulses are
naturally overcome by the child's capacity to play.

In the process of play, there is an optimal relationship between the id, the ego, and superego, between primary and secondary processes. Primary affects are harnessed in play, in that they are tamed and used, rather than subdued. Most 5-year-old little-brother-haters "play out" their rage by dropping or drowning their baby dolls and, later, saving and rescuing them from terrible imaginary fates. In play, these children *retain* their aggressive life and capacity, but their aggression in this form is acceptable to the ego. No real damage is done to the baby brother, because play does not really count and it stands outside reality.

Through play the child develops and retains her fantasy world, her capacity for imagination, and she learns to move comfortably between her inner life and current reality. Gradually, this capacity to play and create is modified and, at times, lost as we become adults and as secondary process thinking and the reality principle hold sway. Adults who retain the capacity to be playful tend to maintain an inner and outer world harmony. People who are humorous and have a capacity for playful metaphor are typically attractive to others. The creative artist usually retains a unique ability to explore his or her internal life and imagination and renders the images encountered to the world at large. The function of play is linked to the eventual capacity for fantasy, imagination and creativity, and the ability to play with ideas (Greenacre, 1971; Plaut, 1979).

DEVELOPMENTAL USAGES

Because play has a special position between the inner and outer worlds it has many development-promoting capacities. The function of play allows a child to think about her actions. For example, the nursery school child takes on the roles of others in play. The child becomes "Mommy" or "Daddy" or "baby," "teacher" or "policeman." In the process she begins to experience what others do, think, and feel. These experiences are important in the process of "decentering," helping the young child move from her narcissistic self to feel what others feel. Play therefore helps children develop this significant capacity for empathy by learning about the people around them.

Moreover, children often master difficult events through play (Waelder, 1933). For example, by concretely using child dolls who are surrounded by play doctors and make-believe hospital equipment, a child can slowly make sense of a hospital experience. An event that was initially conceived as a painful punishment slowly becomes seen as a treatment for a physical problem.

Play also provides a special source of pleasure in dealing with the naturally occurring daily difficulties and "put-downs." Becoming Superman for a half hour after school helps a child overcome the experience of being little and vulnerable, ordered about by parents and teachers. Superman, in play, has a consoling and refueling function.

Because play is pervasive in childhood, it provides an opportunity for immediate connections. It is a universal language among children. The new child on the block typically does not need a long introduction. She knocks on a neighbor child's door and asks, "Do you want to play?" thus achieving a natural entree to the new community.

Many children, particularly those with emotional problems, have difficulties with their capacity to play, and these limits may significantly interfere with their unfolding development.

PLAY AND THE OBJECT TIE

Winnicott(1968) has noted that the capacity to play in childhood is linked to "good enough" object development. Although a capacity for play has an innate component (puppies and kittens are playful), it is clearly developed by the early parent–child relationship and dependent on the early playful object. Most "good enough" parents naturally play with their children throughout the day. A spoonful of cereal becomes an airplane flying into the open mouth; the little "shoezy" wiggles back and forth until it finds the right foot to pounce upon. As the young child builds her connection to mother and father, she simultaneously builds her connection to the function of play. Thus, Winnicott (1968) has observed, most children develop "a play space" to which they are highly attached.

IMPLICATIONS FOR
THE CHILD THERAPIST

Play is the emotional language of the child, and the therapist and the atmosphere of the office should be conducive to the child's play, so that her internal life can unfold. The office should be an open stage, where the child's imagination can be expressed without restraint in an atmosphere that allows her to reveal what she thinks and feels. Such expression differs from "talking to adults," which retains many aspects of a foreign communication that has been learned and used as propaganda and disinformation for adults.

The child therapist must develop the capacity to become a *player*, to "regress in the service of the ego" with the child, to animate and vivify the unfolding material. This capacity forges a major link between child and therapist, and enhances and develops the therapeutic alliance. Internally, the child links the therapist with the early pleasurable playful parent. The child also feels that she is in a special "play space" (Winnicott, 1968)) with someone who can understand and speak her special language. The original object, the parent, communicating effectively with the young child, is there to "enjoy the good, make right the bad, and render the ununderstandable understandable" (Oremland, 1998). Within the "play space" the new object, the therapist, can help to make things comprehensible as the child plays out her internal world. Using the template of the parental object, the therapist can become the person with whom the most fear-laden areas of thought are expressed (Oremland, 1998).

The child's capacity to play has many diagnostic implications. How well and freely does the child patient play? Is she inhibited—is the play frozen, repetitive, or stereotyped? Is the play too impulsive, wild, and out of control? Ideally, play should be a mixture of action and thought. We learn a great deal about a child by observing her play and assessing the child's progress by following the quality of her play during the course of treatment. Can her imaginative, pretending and playful capabilities unfold? Again, because the capacity for imaginative play suggests a harmony between the internal and external life, this is often an important barometer for effective treatment.

Parents need to understand the importance of play in their child's daily life as well as in the therapy hour. On one hand, this will help them appreciate the role of play in the therapy process. But, more important, understanding the parent's capacity for playfulness will tell the therapist a great deal about family life. What are the taboos and restraints within the family? Are there opportunities for pleasurable interaction? Obviously, helping parents and children develop some areas for mutual play may significantly affect the course of treatment by enhancing the parent–child ties.

CLINICAL MATERIAL

In the following case material with Douglas, a 6½-year-old boy, I discuss the preplay and play phases emerging in psychotherapy.

Douglas was a handsome, intelligent, vigorous youngster, the older of two brothers in an intact family. Both parents were professionals and thoughtful individuals. In Douglas's history, his parents stated that he had always been motorically active since birth. During toddlerhood he evidenced impulsive, aggressive behavior. He hit, kicked, bit other children, had temper tantrums, and always needed limits. There seemed to be problems in modulating all affects. In school, he had poor attention, attacked other children, and was easily distracted.

He was diagnosed as a youngster with attention-deficit/hyperactivity disorder (ADHD), and although the use of Ritalin appeared to help somewhat, many problems persisted. In my evaluation, it was clear that he was a counterphobic child who was very frightened internally. He anticipated attackers and punishments, and he handled this by becoming the attacker. The purpose of the treatment was to help Douglas learn of his internal fears and to become more comfortable with them. There was no evidence of particular difficult or traumatic early events in his life. I thought his mother could be somewhat intrusive and controlling at times. Douglas had had a tonsillectomy at age 4, which had exacerbated his difficult behavior for a period of time.

I am going to describe two phases of the early treatment of Douglas: first, a period with little or no play; second, after 5 months, a shift to vigorous play between us.

In the early months of treatment, Douglas was a difficult patient, as many such youngsters are. He was often directly angry with me. He would verbally "slap my face." He was provocative; he turned on the clock radio, put his shoes on the wall, and tried to open the window on the 19th floor (in my office). He used many curse words to see my reaction: "fucker," "motherfucker," "bitch." Often this behavior was accompanied by anxiety, expressed by eye blinking or rocking. He told me that when he became 17 he would be so strong that nobody would mess with him. If I commented that he might be a little scared of me, he yelled that that was a stupid idea coming from a retard.

Any attempt at play was aborted. Douglas might make several ships out of clay, but would quickly break them down. Sometimes bodies emerged out of the clay, and he would use scissors to cut off body parts. But he could tolerate no words about, or even my attention to, what he was doing. Yet in a general way during this period of time, he was becoming more at ease in the office, more comfortable with the toys and the routine, and he smiled at me occasionally when our eyes met.

In this first phase Douglas was not playing with me during these hours. Like the patient Mark (discussed in Chapter 1), he was very frightened of me, and he could not distinguish between his destructive fantasies and the reality of the situation. Because of his projections of aggression onto me (e.g., I would hurt him so he needed to be a strong 17-year-old), he could not get any distance from his internal life.

I describe these early months as a preplay period, when despite no apparent letup of his counterphobic stance, a great deal was happening. Slowly Douglas has gained an opportunity to test his frightening conceptions: Do I live up to his fearful expectation? Over a period of time I do not react to his provocation. I remain consistent and dependable, meeting with him twice weekly for the full number of sessions. I am nonjudgmental; I do not deplore his cursing, but I point out from time to time that he reacts so strongly because he is a little scared of me. In the office I am also an affect regulator. There are many things he can do or say, but he cannot damage toys or furniture, mark the walls, or break things. Despite his intense feeling, the office remains a safe place where much can be expressed within manageable limits.

These elements of our interaction begin to change his relationship with me. He begins to believe I will not hurt him. The office and I are safe; moreover, he is in a unique place where he can express a lot of intense feelings. The ingredients are also available—toys, crayons, and supplies, as well as a playmate—for him to find a creative, new way to express these inside feelings. Douglas then moves to the *play period*.

After about a 5-month period, Douglas told me that he was "Jack the Ripper." I asked him who I was, and he said, "The worry doctor." I wondered how old Jack the Ripper was, and Douglas said, "Eight." Then he added, "I guess I'm Jack the Little Ripper."

Jack and the worry doctor had clay guns, and Jack developed a game. First he knocked on the doctor's door. I asked, "Who is there?" and he said, "Jack the Ripper." I was to act very upset and get my gun to shoot at him. Jack hid behind the chair and shot back. I hid behind the pillow; we fought for a long time.

Now Jack wanted to play every hour, and we took a long preparatory time to fashion our clay guns. They had triggers and sights, bullet cartridges, and even sequins.

During our play, after several vigorous shooting encounters, I would take "time out" to talk. I would comment about the play. I noted that he was worried about a big worry doctor hurting him, and boys his age also worried about big daddies hurting them. He liked to shoot me, and sometimes he had ideas, like all boys, about hurting his daddy.

Although Douglas said nothing to me about his concern, he began to talk to his mother at home. He told her he worried about his dad—his dad was too skinny (his father was having some stomach trouble at the time). Would his dad become very sick? When his father took a trip during this period, Douglas became very anxious; he verbalized to his mother that he feared that his dad would be killed in the airplane. These discussions seemed to relieve Douglas.

In his Jack the Ripper play, Douglas now became quite interested in my elaborate gun. He wanted to shoot it out of my hand. He shot the gun so that it went flying (in the play I had to throw it several feet). He gave it karate chops so that it broke into pieces. He extracted the bullets.

I began to talk in our time-outs about feelings boys had about their daddy's gun, how jealous boys felt because they worried that their own guns were too small. They want at times to break their daddy's gun/penis. Douglas picked up my gun and punched holes in it with a pencil so all the "piss" could come out from everywhere.

At times during this play Douglas felt very guilty. For example, he wanted me to kill Jack the Ripper and riddle him with bullets. I refrained, telling him that all boys had these jealous "ripper" feelings. At home Douglas told his mother and father, "I do bad things . . . you should send me to an orphanage. I don't think when I'm doing things."

Douglas now wanted to come to treatment, and he talked of me in a very affectionate way to his parents. He would say, "I'm going to see my Chethik," or if he passed my office building, he would comment, "This is my Chethik's building. Is he there now?" He was becoming much less a behavior problem both generally and in my office, although he remained a very vigorous youngster.

Characteristically, after our "Jack" play for the day, we played sports. We developed a vigorous basketball game, using a Nerf ball and hoop attached to my door. We constructed "fair rules," so either of us could win with a handicap I had that made the game fair. If Douglas cheated, which was very often, I would comment that we were now using the "Douglas rules" rather than the "what's fair is fair rules."

In our "Jack" games, he was now shooting off parts of my body. Fingernails and thumbs went, and I would need immediate surgery. I began to comment about his tonsillectomy when he was a little boy, and we were able to construct a Tonsillectomy Book. Douglas now decided, after shooting off parts of my body, to play "Jack the Dick Ripper." He would shoot off my penis; I would hold myself, according to his direction, in the crotch area and wail. Jack laughed intensely. I could slowly verbalize again how jealous boys were about worry doctors' and daddies' dicks. Douglas's creative variations continued. After the dick ripper hit its mark, he had my wife enter in play and look aghast at my serious wounds.

In my discussions with him, I knew he was very jealous because now (in reality) his mother was pregnant again. I said this made him feel small and left out. He screamed at me that she wasn't pregnant, she was fat. Eye blinking ensued, and Douglas said he wouldn't let the baby use his toys. He now allowed me to talk for long periods about his jealous feelings, his baby-killing wishes, and so forth, but he kept his eyes closed. When I asked him whether he was asleep he said no, he was in a coma and he wouldn't come out for years.

With this play and my interpretations, we saw less and less acting out in treatment, at home, and at school, and more vigorous sports games, after the Ripper stories, that adhered to the "what's fair is fair rules." Douglas could lose at times in basketball with some grace.

How can we understand the *play relationship* that developed between Douglas and his therapist? Two aspects emerged simultaneously. One component is the *transference relationship*. Clearly, the "worry doctor" is a displacement for the father. Combat with the feared, castrating father is lived out in the son's play. Jealousy and castration themes are very evident. The phallic–oedipal conflict is played out and verbalized, and significant aspects of the conflict are worked through.

A second and critical component of the play relationship is the *therapeutic alliance*, the play relationship that develops between the two players. Not only is Douglas invested in the content (the oedipal struggle), but he comes to love the process and the developing enactment of his internal story. The therapist becomes "my Chethik." There is a growing, loving tie to the therapist.

I am suggesting that the therapist and Douglas have recreated the transitional *play space* that Winnicott (1968) described. The therapist is not only the bad worry doctor in the transference, but also the special person who plays, explores, discovers, and elicits ideas. Douglas becomes creative in the relationship: Jack the Ripper, Jack the Little Ripper, Jack the Dick Ripper. He is an author unfolding new scenes and chapters.

Why does the alliance develop? What is the therapist's contribution? In the play situation the therapist is especially attuned to the child's internal life. Initially he becomes an enthusiastic player under the child's direction, living out the scenes of the child's internal life. Second, through the therapist's empathy and understanding he can verbalize and clarify the child's inner turmoil. Over the months of regular work with regular appointments the therapist also becomes a consistent, available and enduring object on which the child can rely. The therapist also functions as an affect regulator; he can allow the emergence of intense and important affects, but simultaneously erects a safe atmosphere so that these affects are not overwhelming and flooding.

These qualities of therapy—empathy, consistency, availability, affect regulation, opportunities for creative expression through play—foster the libidinal aspect of the alliance and form the context in which interpretative work can occur. This attachment has its history in the early "good enough" relationship between parent and child and their early libidinal play.

What are the curative aspects of this interplay? Douglas's acting out diminishes generally. The interpretative work is important. Douglas has "ripper feelings" toward his dad. When his primitive aggressive feelings are verbalized, accepted, and normalized, this fosters structural change within Douglas. The harshness of his superego reactions and the intensity of his guilt diminish, because he has learned that he has ideas that all growing boys share. Another critical change component stems from the play relationship and should be understood in object relations terms. The therapist welcomes Douglas's internal life, which unfolds through the play. His inside ideas, his mind, is valuable. Just as the young child feels that his worth is enhanced when his mother approves of his creative productions, Douglas finds and experiences an accepting regard for his material and elaborated productions.

In this chapter, I have focused on the role of play in work with children. There is a growing recognition that play in a large sense, has an important role in adult psychotherapy (Benveniste, 1998; London, 1981). Sanville (1991), in her book *The Playground of Psychoanalytic Therapy*, describes how therapy becomes a playground where needs and wishes and versions of oneself that are yearned for

can be expressed and explored. In an effective treatment both therapist and patient need to experience the importance of play and illu-
sion in human life.

BIBLIOGRAPHY

Benveniste, D. (1998). The importance of play in adulthood. *Psychoanalytic Study of the Child* 53:51–64.

Greenacre, P. (1971). Play in relation to creative imagination. In: *Emotional Growth*, Vol. II. New York: International Universities Press.

London, N. (1981). The play element of regression in the psychoanalytic process. *Psychoanalytic Inquiry*, Vol. 1, no. 1, 7–27. New York: International Univer-sities Press.

Mayes, S., & Cohen, D. (1993). Playing and therapeutic action in child analysis. *International Journal of Psycho-Analysis*. 73:1235–1244.

Oremland, J. (1998). Play, dreams and creativity. *Psychoanalytic Study of the Child*. 53:84–93.

Plaut, E. (1979). Play and adaptation. *Psychoanalytic Study of the Child*. 34:217–232.

Scott, M. (1998). Play and therapeutic action. *Psychoanalytic Study of the Child*. 53:94–101.

Shengold, L. (1988). Comments on play. *Bulletin of the Anna Freud Clinic*. 11, Part 2: 146–151.

Sanville, J. (1991). *The Playground of Psychoanalytic Therapy*. Hillsdale, NJ: The Analytic Press.

Waelder, R. (1933). The psychoanalytic theory of play. *Psychoanalytic Quarterly*. 2:208–224.

Winnicott, D. (1968). Playing: Its theoretical status in the clinical situation. *International Journal of Psycho-Analysis*. 49:591–598.

II

~

Work with Parents

Introduction

An area that has received relatively little attention in child psychotherapy is work with parents. It is obvious that no child in treatment
can prosper without the sanction of his parents, and it is the parental
support of the treatment that *allows* the child to use the therapy experience.

In Part II we look at a range of interventions with parents, which
include the following:

1. Parent guidance
2. Transference parenting
3. Treatment of the parent–child relationship

Typically, one begins all parent work with "parent guidance."
Parent guidance is primarily an educational form of intervention, and
varied aspects are discussed in Chapter 4. The premise in this form of
work is that treatment tasks will be faciliated by an effective alliance
between the therapist (his treatment goals for the child) and the parents (their healthy, adaptive capacities).

At times, however, there are problems in parent work because of
limits within the parents. Some parents who are relatively more disturbed and dependent make better use of the intervention of "transference parenting" (also described in Chapter 4). This form of intervention provides the "sustenance" that some parents need, and this is
fully described in this section.

There are also many parents who consciously want to help their child, but whose child has some major unconscious meaning for them that fosters the pathology and difficulties in the child. The technique of "treatment of the parent–child relationship" can be utilized to provide some insight, so that the parent can interact with the child in a less encumbered way. Chapter 5 illustrates this process and discusses some of the difficulties and limits. The work with parents is further illustrated, elaborated, and discussed throughout the book in Parts III and IV.

4

~

Parent Guidance and
Transference Parenting

In this chapter two approaches with parents are discussed—the techniques of *parent guidance* and, later, the process of *transference parenting*. The initial and most common approach with parents is parent guidance. This process assumes that the parent has relatively good ego functioning and that he or she identifies with the goals of the treatment. Basically, it is supportive work.

In the literature on parent work, authors describe a wide spectrum of issues that they subsume under parent guidance. Sandler, Kennedy, and Tyson (1980) have discussed general goals. They see the function of parent guidance as a process to ensure providing continuing emotional and practical support" to the child treatment. In addition, this work should "lend support to the parent's self-esteem." Arnold (1978) describes parent guidance as a continuum from simple information or education through advice, permission, and clarification, depending on what is necessary. Weisberger (1986) also specifies a number of goals and processes. Parent guidance should mobilize the familial environment to support better parental functioning, thereby relieving unrealistic and unhealthy pressures on the child. In addition, she notes that parent guidance should offer information about growth and development and give practical help

Steven Rubin, psychology intern, provided some of the clinical material used in this chapter.

with management. All of these authors imply that parent guidance is not an interpretative process. Essentially, the therapist works with parents' conscious or preconscious material.

Because there are a large variety of issues that are welcomed in parent guidance, we suggest two general categories as broad domains for parent guidance work and list specific areas of work within each category:

1. Issues that affect the emotional balance in the family, which include:
   a. Working with general difficulties in either parent's life that may affect his or her ability to parent.
   b. Working on differences between parents regarding the handling of their children.
   c. Working with stresses that emerge in parents caused by the fact that their child is in treatment (e.g., a sense of failure, fear of the child's attachment to the therapist, etc.).
2. Issues that center on the child patient primarily, which include:
   a. Receiving from the parents current reality information about child and family events.
   b. Imparting to the parents a *general* understanding of child development and the internal affective life of the child.
   c. Imparting to the parents a *specific* understanding of the child patient's symptoms or behavior changes that emerge (the purpose is to help parents cope with the behaviors or symptoms or with the changes that emerge within treatment).
   d. Clarification with parents of the problematic interactions between themselves and the child patient (the purpose is to alter parental handling by highlighting the interactions, advising changes, and providing explanations for the changes).

The following clinical examples illustrate the varieties and dimensions of parent guidance work.

CASE 1

Nathan was a 6½-year-old "hellion" who had evidenced many problems in kindergarten and first grade in public school because of his aggressive behavior with peers. Children and teachers became concerned at the intensity of his rage, which was primarily promoted (we learned in the course of his therapy) by his underlying fears of punishment.

There had been a divorce in the family when Nathan was 3, and this event had prompted a good deal of difficulty. Nathan and his mother appeared to have an enmeshed relationship that was troubling for him, and he also felt responsible for having "driven" his father away. The parents had joint custody, in terms of both decision making and physical custody. The therapist saw the parents separately, inasmuch as mutual animosity made joint meetings impossible.

Much of the early work centered on the difficulties with effective discipline in both houses. Very often, Nathan simply would not comply (e.g., climbing on furniture, refusing bedtime, coming to dinner late). It became clear that both parents felt a need to "cater" to him, to give in to him. His mother wondered whether he was "fragile," and his father tended to look the other way, waiting until he went back to his other home. Slowly both parents, in examining some of their motives for laxity, realized they felt a great deal of guilt about the impact of the divorce on their youngster. They felt that they had caused him enough suffering, and that they were the source of his pain. With this internal understanding, and the evidence that the problems in discipline at home fostered difficulties in the community for their son, both parents developed more effective standards. This went beyond the demands for compliance and involved appropriate responsibility for a youngster his age—helping to fold his clothing and putting laundry away, getting his own glass of water, and so forth.

As some of the divorce issues were traced, both parents discussed their rage and frustration with each other following the divorce. The father described how he used to hate to answer the telephone—the mother would be calling to berate him and issue yet another demand. The mother lamented her lost opportunities because of the divorce. She had supported her husband through his advanced schooling years, and they had had an understanding that she would have a similar opportunity. Now, because of economics, there was no free future. She generally felt that the burdens of being a single parent were more difficult for her to bear because of her relative financial constriction. The effect of this bitter unloading of the past (done in individual sessions) allowed the parents to work more freely together around Nathan's issues.

A major additional theme in the work in the first year with the parents was helping them to understand the implications for an "oedipal" child in the aftermath of a divorce. The therapist was aware that Nathan was struggling with the oedipal phase of development by virtue of his age, while simultaneously dealing with the separation and divorce in his family. Two major features of the normal oedipal phase would have to be kept in mind: (1) the affectionate and sexualized relationship with the mother and (2) the heightened competitive relationship and rivalry with the father. The mother brought up Nathan's "touching" problem, which she had previously wanted to avoid. Nathan had sought to kiss her on the lips or "accidentally" fondle her breasts. The therapist's general discussion of the intense natural sexuality of children and how it is enhanced when there is no prohibiting father allowed the mother to gain some perspective on Nathan's "excitement problem." She could also, then, use the information to take more appropriate steps with modesty. For example, she would now have Nathan take his own bath because he needed "privacy."

When Nathan's mother broke off a year-long relationship with her boyfriend, Nathan was very upset for a number of weeks. The therapist noted that her relationship had made Nathan feel safer in the house—it had inhibited some of his excitement urges. When his mother spoke to Nathan, he intensely related his worry that he "drives everyone away— his daddy also."

Another general theme in the parent guidance was the identification of underlying issues when a crisis of aggression emerged in school. For example, on one occasion Nathan had been very aggressive toward several boys in his class for a number of days. "Randy almost tore my arm off," "Joshua made a deep cut on my arm," complained Nathan. When the therapist explored this behavior with his parents, it emerged that his paternal grandfather had recently had emergency surgery on an embolism that was lodged in a vein in his leg. This had aroused much anxiety within the child. With encouragement, the father spoke to his son about the operation. Nathan voiced a number of anxieties: "Will grandpa die?" "Will they have to cut his leg off?" When these concerns could be addressed realistically, Nathan slept peacefully for the first time in a week. After the discussion the fighting in school abated.

Discussion

This material illustrates a number of features of parent guidance work. One aspect is *dealing with the typical problems of adults that can interfere with their effective parenting*. Both of Nathan's parents are relatively well integrated individuals who clearly identified with the goals of Nathan's treatment and who functioned well generally in their lives. The divorce, however, had left many residual scars that interfered with their parenting capacities at times. Both parents felt very guilty about the disruption in their child's life and tried to make up to Nathan by minimizing his frustration and avoiding setting limits. His mother also, at times, partly made up for her own loneliness by an unduly intense attachment to her son. When these patterns were noted, the parents could respond effectively. In addition, because of the past bitterness in their relationship, they found it hard to work conjointly regarding their son. The opportunity for some discharge of feelings, stemming from the impact of their failed relationship on their later adjustment, allowed them to put the past somewhat in perspective.

Another component of parent guidance is the therapist's ability to *generally describe the internal life of the child* so that the parents can gain greater awareness of the developmental process. A major theme in the preceding material was sorting out with the parents the underlying oedipal dynamics particularly affected by a divorce. The therapist highlighted the typical sexuality of a 6½-year-old boy and his exaggerated fears of impulse expression without the inhibiting father. This glimpse of the internal erotic struggles of Nathan alerted his mother to the need for more physical distance from her son, as well as far greater privacy and modesty, and helped her understand his strong reactions to her male friends. These dynamics also helped the child's father to become the "heavy" with Nathan (he could be the prohibitor), which was a role he had until now avoided.

The therapist also helped the parents to *understand some of the patient's specific dynamics*, another aspect of parent guidance work. Nathan was a counterphobic youngster—when he became frightened (often projected fears) he "identified with the aggressor" and often lashed out. Castration anxiety was a major theme in the direct work with Nathan. There were many opportunities to help the parents understand that when Nathan became aggressive (manifest behavior), he was often frightened internally. Thus, the therapist and parents could clearly trace Nathan's attacks and worries about his arm to the surgery of his grandfather. Their growing ability, in the course of treatment, to help Nathan understand the "scary" roots to his hellionlike behavior outbursts enhanced the overall therapeutic process.

CASE 2

Andrew was a 12-year-old whose parents became concerned because of an exacerbation of problems about 6 months before they came for evaluation. He appeared to have become acutely depressed, expressed constant dissatisfaction with himself, and avoided investing very much in his schoolwork because he was "shattered by the errors" he naturally made in the course of his work. The evaluation underscored that Andrew was a neurotic youngster. The primary dynamics seemed to center on unresolved oedipal conflicts, particularly a struggle with his competitive and phallic feelings emerging from his relationship to his father.

In the conjoint work with both parents, an important focus was the father's anger with his son. After a period of time, Mr. J, a business executive who commanded a large work force, acknowledged that he had an anger problem—he had high standards for himself and his children, and he was "quick on the trigger" at times and aware of his explosiveness. Thus, part of Andrew's difficulty in his competitive feelings with his father and others stemmed from an external problem—the father's demandingness and anger that evoked counter-rage and fear in his son.

Because the father cared about his son and identified with the goals of the treatment, he slowly became increasingly able to observe his interactions with his son; he also permitted both the therapist and his wife to explore these events. In board and card games at home, the father had instinctively pressed his son for better performance and was aware of his own angry countenance. When Andrew was having problems with math and had difficulty with his father's tutoring, Mr. J had yelled, "You WILL learn to do this now!" and his son had broken into tears. The father began to observe and evaluate how he had reacted when there had been minor "transgressions"—when his son's manners slipped, or when his son interrupted him momentarily when he was working on the computer, for example. He became increasingly aware of the tension and anger these experiences with his son evoked. He spoke of his own mother's ridicule and demeaning behavior toward him throughout his own childhood years and felt that in some ways he was repeating this type of behavior.

As the father became more fully aware of his patterns, he discussed with his son his own temper problem after some outbursts, and at times apologized for his overreactions. At first Andrew responded with intense anger: "You are never satisfied with me—I hate you!!" At times, depression was evident—"You are much smarter, and I'm dumb." But after a period of an ongoing life-space dialogue, Andrew began to develop some humor and distance from his own counter-rage. After losing in checkers to his father, Andrew mused, "I hate your guts again, but you didn't beat me by too much." The father began to take his son to work on occasion to show him some aspects of his work environment, and he also told his son that a motor bike stored in the back of the shed would become his when he reached driving age. They would rebuild it together. Generally, the father became able to modify his reactions of rage against his son significantly and to acknowledge his overreactions when they emerged.

Discussion

The clinical process with the J's occurred over the course of a year, while Andrew was in the process of psychotherapy. *One facet of parent guidance work is the process of helping parents become aware of aspects of themselves and their handling of their youngsters that unfavorably affect their child's development.* Although Andrew had internalized conflicts, one component of his depression/self-hatred was the external conflict with his father.

As a trusting relationship developed between the therapist and the parents, the therapist could identify this angry, harsh feature between father and son, as emanating from the father. Although such confrontations are always threatening to parents, Mr. J had the capacity to accept this aspect of himself and follow it closely in the course of the work. Mr. J was an effective individual within his profession and family and had the capacity for self-observation. He also clearly wanted to help remedy the difficulties his son had developed; he had, as well, an appropriate measure of guilt regarding his earlier interactions with his son. The "exposure" of these interactions with his son did not evoke the intense humiliation (and defensive denials) that we often see in parents with narcissistic problems.

In the course of the year, Mr. J was able to significantly master and modify his pathogenic interactions with his son. His self-awareness (ego awareness) led him to become conscious of the situations that evoked his rage with his son and of the quality of his overreactions (as it was necessary for him to continue to limit his child appropriately). This monitoring process had an important effect on their interactions. Mr. J did not need insight (to understand the unconscious meaning that his son represented) in order to make this change. Although he commented that the situation represented a part of his own childhood, this aspect was not fully explored. The parent guidance process made explicit a pattern of interaction that Mr. J was aware of on a preconscious level. If greater internal understanding had been necessary for the change, the appropriate intervention would have been a form of "treatment of the parent–child relationship," which is explored in the next chapter.

CASE 3

Gerald was 11 years old at the time of his evaluation; he was a member of an intact middle-class family and the second sibling in a sibship of four. He was the only boy. He had been referred for his generally "obnoxious" behavior. Nothing seemed to please him, and he felt any task or demand was "unfair." He was sullen about taking out the garbage and complained to his parents when his day was not interesting enough. He was arrogant with his few friends, bossing and ridiculing them. Although he was bright, he found his homework "boring," did few assignments in school, and acted like a clown in class.

In the early work with Gerald's parents, his mother appeared particularly anxious. Her "schedule" made it hard for the parents to show up on time for their sessions. She eyed the therapist with suspicion, seemed eager to leave quickly, and wrung her hands or talked volubly and intensely. She wondered on several occasions what her son had had to say about her in his sessions. When the therapist noted some of these signs of discomfort, she acknowledged her sense of apprehension. Would the therapist find something wrong with her? He commented that parents are often concerned they have contributed to difficulties and then approach the therapy with worry that they will be criticized.

Mrs. A confessed, as therapy commenced, that she feared she had spoiled her son. She guessed that she had tended to do too much for him. She found herself catering to his needs in a way she did not with her daughters. She always asked him what special foods he wanted included in his lunch and complied with his requests to be driven wherever he wanted to go. She was anxious about these confessions—"Have I hurt him?" "Is he too spoiled?" The therapist pointed out that she herself seemed already to have an awareness that Gerald generally had trouble tolerating frustration, and her need to give into him was probably not helpful. The mother noted that she found it hard to stand the anger he would express, and she was always worried about him.

This general apprehension about her son had other manifestations. Gerald tended to complain about his body (neck pains or leg pains), and Mrs. A quickly had to check with the family pediatrician. In addition, when her husband (a rather passive and busy man) attempted to impose some limits, she invariably defended her son and found mitigating circumstances for the least transgression. Thus, the sanction was never imposed. When the therapist underscored the problems she had in imposing effective limits, Mrs. A acknowledged her role in the sessions. She feared that she could become too angry and had impulses to send Gerald to a military school. ("Does this mean I'm a very bad mother?" she would interpose anxiously.) She knew that in the past, as she grew up, she had been very angry with her brother. She wondered whether that could be affecting her relationship with her son.

Despite the somewhat driven quality of her need to protect and overindulge her son, the awareness of these patterns mobilized Mrs. A to alter her approach. With the major support of her husband, routines and rules were established. Allowance was curtailed for mishaps, a bedtime schedule was established, study time was enforced, and Gerald was effectively sent to his room for his "obnoxious" outbursts and argumentativeness. During the weekly meetings with the therapist, Mrs. A commented on her continued internal anxiety and her apprehension after she had set limits. However, she felt a great deal of relief when Gerald's schoolwork improved and he responsibly ran a paper route for a 6-month period.

Discussion

In the preceding parent guidance work, Mrs. A had rather typical reactions at the start of treatment. *Bringing their youngster for treatment often evokes a myriad of reactions by parents.* Most parents experience a sense of failure when they acknowledge that their child has emotional problems. They often feel internally responsible for the difficulties. Whereas some parents handle their guilt initially by attacking the therapist (they fear condemnation), many anxiously "confess," as did Mrs. A. When the "expert" therapist can tolerantly acknowledge some contribution to the difficulties the child has, without the attack they fear, parents often feel a good deal of relief.

Many parents have a preconscious idea about problems in handling their children, as we have seen in the case of Mr. J. Mrs. A was quite aware of her need to cater, indulge, and overidentify with her son. The process of parent guidance allowed her to make these patterns more ego-distonic (alien to her) and to take concrete steps to better her handling. Earlier she had used many rationalizations to continue "protecting" her son. As in the other case illustrations, the healthy aspects of Mrs. A's ego allowed her to mobilize techniques to effectively frustrate and limit this youngster. Although she wondered about the early sources for the difficulty in handling (e.g., her relationship with her brother), this was not a central area of work. There was no insight to her past that illuminated this tendency. Rather, her own enhanced self-observation and her desire to help her son fostered the changes in her daily interactions with him.

CASE 4

Rita was an attractive, well-dressed, but somewhat stocky 5-year-old at the time of evaluation. Her parents had brought her for therapy because of her increasing sense of panic when she separated from her mother, an inability to become "unfrozen" in nursery school, and a generalized stubborness and anger that permeated her demeanor. In the past year there had also been a steady weight gain. Rita had two older brothers (one brother, Robert, was just 1½ years older than she), and there was also a new sibling, Tanya, who was only 6 months of age. Both parents had a professional background, and the father was particularly busy and preoccupied at work inasmuch he was struggling to achieve tenure in an academic setting. The evaluation revealed that Rita was struggling with two levels of conflict: pre-oedipal anger that had been evident in her toilet training history and expressed in her current stubborness; and penis envy issues that particularly focused on her next oldest brother, Robert. Rita was seen twice weekly, and her parents were seen conjointly every other week. The parents were highly motivated to help their daughter and understand their own influences on her development, and they also seemed to have a good, mutually supportive relationship.

In the early phases of the parent work, Mrs. D became aware of the enormous sense of burden she felt raising this large "nest of children." Although there was often much pleasure, she was quite overwhelmed by the sheer level of the daily demands, the endless tasks, and the fact that her day never seemed to end. At times, she cried unexpectedly toward the end of the day and often felt extremely fatigued. Was she depressed, she wondered? Much affect emerged when she discussed her promising past professional career. She had indeed had a very stimulating, high-paying job after college in which she had clearly been highly valued. Currently, on occasion, her former boss came by with some task or problem, which she handled on a consultative basis. The contrast to the daily "drudgery" began further to explain the fatigue and sense of depletion she experienced from time to time. She laughed when she noted that her work at home was not terribly intellectually stimulating. This general discussion began to provide a thoughtful framework for Mrs. D. She could now understand her periods of intermittent depression, although she clearly also loved being a mother. At times she had felt she was endlessly trapped by diapers, but she began to realize that as her tasks abated (as the children moved into school) she could slowly renew her professional contacts and interests.

Mrs. D had also made few demands on her husband for child-rearing as his career had reached a critical juncture. But it emerged that Professor D was often only a "play daddy." For example, when he came home late in the evening (a number of times per week), he took several of the children out of bed, because he missed them. The excitement and stimulation undid the sleep preparation routine, and chaos could ensue for another hour. Mrs. D was internally very resentful, but she also felt that the children and father needed each other. These discussions began to highlight the lack of support the mother felt she received from her husband, in areas of discipline, routine, and general child care. The father noted humorously that perhaps this explained some of his wife's sexual withdrawal at times when she said, "I'm too tired." The couple began to make changes that were mutually agreeable—for example, father could come home for dinner every night, spend time with the children, help "bed them down," and then return to the office. But he realized he could also bring certain of his work tasks home.

At times, Mrs. D observed that she had felt tense with Rita and a sense of alienation. She did not experience this with the other children, and this distance upset her. As we looked at the weekly incidents, a pattern emerged. Mrs. D would stay in the bedroom with Rita saying goodnight until Rita "allowed" her to leave. At times, she felt estranged when Rita was talking very loudly and angrily to her. It became clear that Mrs. D had a good deal of difficulty in firmly limiting and making demands on her daughter. We found that Rita had virtually no chores, whereas the older boys worked appropriately within the house. Mrs. D preconsciously anticipated any potentially difficult confrontation with her "stubborn" daughter and worked assiduously to circumvent a blow-up. She also feared, the therapist noted, her own anger toward her daughter. All agreed that the demands, frustrations, and blow-ups were necessary, and it was underscored that if she became less afraid of her child's emerging anger, this would be a reassurance to her daughter. Mrs. D became increasingly able to insist that Rita work with her around dinner preparation, setting the table, and so forth, and she did not "give in" to Rita's protests when she left her in the bedroom after a reasonable "tucking" in.

Throughout the work with Rita, certain behaviors were highlighted at home as they became an internal focus within the child's psychotherapy. During a particular period of work, Rita's demand for food and stealing of food became prominent. The parents worried further about weight gain—should they put her on a diet, should they lock the cupboards? The therapist indicated the natural feelings all children have in relation to siblings: they often feel deprived when there is a new baby and feel (often imagined) and that they are thrown out by the mother. Food becomes a source of solace, because it brings the feeding mother back. Mrs. D then recounted some of the current subtle aggression toward the baby that Rita exhibited. Rita held the baby and hugged her too hard, or the mother would find a penny in the crib that Rita "accidentally" left there. Mrs. D was a resourceful and intuitive mother; in her next appointment she described a new game she had played with Rita. When she was diapering Tanya, Rita had begun some baby talk. Rather than discourage this or react with guilt as she had earlier done, she entered into a game with "baby Rita." She cooed back to her, made believe she fed her with a spoon, and so on. Rita loved the opportunity for temporary regression, in play she renewed the baby status she had lost, and the rapport between mother and child was reconnected.

Discussion

In this case the parent guidance work had a wide scope. Several factors initially had interfered with Mrs. D's parenting capacity at this stage of her life. The sheer burden of raising four relatively young children and the inability to mourn the loss (perhaps temporary) of her profession were contributing to her feelings of fatigue and despair. It was very helpful to Mrs. D to become aware of her internal struggle—the trapped feelings she had in rearing her children and her rage toward the "play daddy" father who was busy and preoccupied. Whereas clarification of this internal stress was helpful to the parents in making direct changes in the mother's life (having the father more available, structuring time when the mother could be away, etc.), it also "normalized" the negative feelings that Mrs. D experienced at times with her children. She came to feel significantly less burdened by her difficulties and did not need to give unremittingly to her children.

It became clear in the course of the treatment with Rita that a factor contributing to Rita's problems with anger was the difficulty Mrs. D had in allowing herself to experience natural anger toward her daughter. This internal difficulty within the mother exacerbated Rita's own rage and her anxiety about her aggression. She felt unsafe and feared her impulses. One part of the parent guidance was to make Mrs. D *aware of her own problem and how it affected her handling of her daughter*. As this became evident to Mrs. D, through her inability to limit the goodnight rituals, provide demands through chores, and so on, she confronted these issues. Despite her internal apprehension, she faced her daughter's tantrums and rage in response to her demands for help around the house. In this form of parent guidance, Mrs. D did not explore her history, the origin of her fears, the particular reasons Rita was singled out for the mother's anxiety. Within the limits of parent guidance, a preconscious problem had been identified, and this awareness mobilized the healthy ego of the mother to take necessary steps in her daily interactions with her child.

Another theme in the parent work was helping the D's to *understand the internal life of their child* as she struggled with various issues in treatment. Behavior in the child patient can often reflect intensified internal issues that are emerging in the psychotherapy. As Rita's jealousy of her younger sister became intensified, her need to overeat (and themes of food in therapy) became more prominent. Parents often have a need to act, to do something, to deal with an emerging symptom or behavior problem. An important component of parent guidance is to provide parents with a perspective that explains what their youngster is struggling with internally. Thus, the therapist explained Rita's rivalry with the younger sister who had usurped the "baby role" in the family, and the oral regression that was an attempt to deal with these feelings. The parents were able to empathize with Rita's strife, became less anxious about the immediate behavior, and allowed other forms of playful regression in the home (baby talk and play feeding) that circumvented Rita's need to overeat.

TRANSFERENCE PARENTING

There are many parents who, either because of early disturbances in their own lives or because of acute current stresses, need further support beyond parent guidance in their work with the child therapist. In some cases, the therapist acts and functions as a nurturing parent to the troubled adult, and this "sustenance" allows the parent to provide more adequately for his or her child. I have termed this process "transference parenting." This also is a form of supportive work, and the following case illustrates this technique.

Clinical Material

Barbara was 6 years of age when she came for outpatient psychotherapy because of a history of severe enuresis. Barbara had been seen for approximately 1 year by her first therapist, Mr. B, in twice-weekly individual play therapy sessions. In addition, Mr. B had met with both of Barbara's parents for weekly parent guidance sessions. Near the end of the first year of Barbara's treatment, Mr. and Mrs. S had decided to separate. Her parents' separation took its toll on Barbara, and she became listless and depressed. In addition, her enuresis (which had lessened to a great extent over the course of the year) became severe once again. At about this time, Mr. B had announced that he would be leaving the agency, and Barbara was faced with coping with two major losses (her father and her therapist) in close succession. Mr. B arranged for a transfer, stipulating that a male therapist was strongly indicated.

This therapist's work with Barbara quickly became divorce focused. In this case, the usual postdivorce adjustment problems were intensified by Mr. S's decision to stop visiting his daughter. Barbara was devastated, and her treatment was utilized to help her cope with the massive rejection and abandonment she felt.

At the point at which he and his wife were separated, Mr. S had stopped attending appointments with Mr. B. Several attempts to engage Mr. S in his daughter's treatment with the new therapist did not prove fruitful. Consequently, the parent work was restricted to sessions with Barbara's mother.

Given her parents' separation, her father's rejection, and the loss of her previous therapist, Barbara was quite an emotionally needy girl. Although it was evident that she would need a great deal of support from her mother, it became equally clear that Mrs. S was terribly needy herself. When the new therapist began working with Mrs. S, she was still feeling the stresses produced by the breakup of her marriage and the demands of being a single parent with little social, emotional, or financial support.

In addition to the current stresses, Mrs. S was also struggling with intense feelings and conflicts toward her own mother, which dated back to her childhood. She described her mother as a "dictator" who had run the household and the lives of those in it. She remembered her father as having been a passive man, "too weak" to leave a miserable marriage. Mrs. S recalled repeated episodes of humiliation and physical abuse at the hands of her mother. She explained that she had received no affection from her parents, resulting in her difficulty in expressing affection to her own child. Recalling her childhood, Mrs. S claimed, "I never learned how to show love."

The clinical dilemma was to find a way to support Mrs. S in such a way that she would better be able to give the love and emotional support her daughter needed from her. A pattern emerged naturally and rather quickly in the sessions with Mrs. S, which turned out to be very productive. In the first part of her sessions, Mrs. S would voice her concerns and worries and describe the struggles that pertained by and large to her own life. Included were her difficulties at work and school (she was working full-time and attending classes at the university), with finances, her relationship to her own parents, feelings about her ex-husband, and, more generally, the trials and tribulations of being a single parent. Mrs. S often began sessions in an agitated state. The therapist would listen, empathize, and offer support. This appeared to have a calming and relieving effect on her. She then was able to move on in the second part of the sessions to focus on issues having more to do with Barbara. At this point, the therapist was able to do some effective parent guidance work that included advice and education concerning child development and Barbara's emotional needs. With time, Mrs. S became increasingly able to put some of the therapist's suggestions into practice effectively as she learned to better parent her daughter. In sum, an effective two-step process had been established whereby the therapist would support and parent Mrs. S so that she, in turn, could better parent and support her daughter.

Several examples help to demonstrate this type of work with parents. When the therapist began working with Mrs. S, she had been working full time and had just reenrolled at the university in order to complete her bachelor's degree. She was quite anxious about her return to school and was able to link some of her worry to her past school failure. Approximately 10 years before, she had begun her undergraduate work in chemistry but found the program too demanding, and she had dropped out in her junior year. She was concerned that she would fail once again. The sessions not only relieved some of her anxiety about her own schoolwork, but they also enabled her to discuss Barbara's academic problems at school. (Barbara's school performance had deteriorated throughout the year following her parents' separation and her father's rejection.) Mrs. S was prone to overidentify with her daughter's problems at school, and the therapist helped her differentiate her own problems and needs from those of her daughter. In this way power struggles between mother and daughter around homework assignments were reduced, and Mrs. S was able to act on the therapist's suggestion that she work closely with her daughter's teacher in order to set clear and reasonable academic expectations for Barbara.

During the first few months postseparation, Mr. S had visited with Barbara on a regular basis. When he then stopped visiting, Mrs. S first had to deal with her own anger and disappointment. In the therapy sessions she was able to verbalize how much she had come to expect and look forward to some free time on the weekends when visitation took place. Once her own disappointment was addressed, Mrs. S became better able to understand and help Barbara with her missing father and hurt feelings. Similarly, when Mrs. S expressed her own ambivalent feel-ings as her divorce was finalized and she anticipated the first Christmas without her ex-husband, she was better able to appreciate Barbara's in-tense sense of loss. The therapist could then work closely with her on making sure that she kept Barbara posted on important events such as the legalization of the divorce and plans as to how the Christmas holiday would be spent.

When Mr. S stopped visiting his daughter altogether, Mrs. S became upset when she felt that Barbara blamed her for her father's actions. Again, once she was able to vent her worries and feelings, she became more supportive and available to Barbara. For example, with the thera-pist's coaching she began to label the "big problems Barbara's father had in being a good daddy."

School, particularly around exam time, was an area that continued to provide a great deal of stress for Mrs. S. Initially, the therapist helped support her through these difficult periods and eventually to anticipate them together ahead of time. This process in itself helped make the stress more manageable. Mrs. S also learned to appreciate that there would be times when she was more or less available to Barbara and to plan ac-cordingly. For example, she was able to explain to Barbara that she was busier during her final exams but that once they were over, the two could do something special together.

Throughout the therapeutic work, the sessions provided "booster shots" that helped Mrs. S to cope with the demands of everyday living, particularly the excessive demands of single parenthood. That she had come to utilize the sessions in this way became quite evident whenever a session was missed because of holiday or illness. Mrs. S would inevitably note the long time between sessions and eagerly and enthusiastically bring the therapist up to date on the events in her own life before turning to issues more focused on Barbara.

After receiving her regular "booster shots" from the therapist, Mrs. S was able to make good use of the advice and suggestions as to how she could be most helpful to Barbara. She became increasingly understand-ing of Barbara's individual psychology and more sensitive to her daugh-ter's emotional needs. Mrs. S was particularly supportive of Barbara in helping her cope with the serious feelings of rejection by her father. Mrs. S, in fact, was able to overcome her own anger, resentment, and bitter-ness in order to support her daughter in her desire to have a relationship with her father. Mrs. S followed many of the therapist's suggestions to explain the divorce to Barbara, to accentuate that Barbara was not at fault or to blame, and, most important, to let her daughter know that she understood how much she missed her father. Mrs. S reported a par-ticularly touching moment with her daughter soon after her father had rejected Barbara's Valentine heart. On a cold, wintery evening, Barbara had gone out on her front porch and started crying. When Mrs. S went to find out what was wrong, Barbara had said, "Nobody loves me." Mrs. S became increasingly available and adept at listening to and acknowledging her daughter's painful feelings.

In addition, Mrs. S was supportive and helpful in Barbara's attempts to reach out and connect with her father. She helped Barbara to write letters, bought presents with her for her father at Christmas and his birthday, and helped arrange for regular visitation with many of her ex-husband's relatives, particularly the paternal grandparents. Although it was difficult at times to secure information as to the whereabouts and goings on of Mr. S, Mrs. S did her best to find out what she could and to pass the information on to Barbara. Mrs. S was also helpful in anticipating potential disappointments for Barbara, especially around her birthday and major holidays.

Throughout a good portion of the 2½ years of working together, Mrs. S appeared to depend heavily on the therapist in these sessions in order to relieve some of her own anxieties and stress and, in turn, to work on her parenting of Barbara. During the last 6 months of treatment, she began to show some signs of growing independence from the therapist. Some of the positive steps she took with Barbara were now initiated on her own and no longer necessarily directly followed discussions in the sessions. For example, one day in a session with Barbara the therapist interpreted her worry that her father might have to go to jail for not paying child support. Barbara responded by saying "I'm not worried because my mom told me she would tell me as soon as she knew, even if it was bad news."

When termination was discussed with Mrs. S, she seemed to feel rather pleased at the progress Barbara had made. The therapist agreed that Barbara had done significant work in dealing with her father's rejection while still maintaining hope that her father would become more available in the future. Barbara's school performance had improved significantly, and she became involved in numerous age-appropriate activities such as cheerleading, learning the recorder, and earning a part in a school play. Her depressive affect had lifted, and obvious gains in self-confidence and self-esteem had been made. Despite periodic enuretic episodes, Mrs. S felt confident that it was time for her daughter's treatment to terminate.

The doubts that surfaced during the termination phase were those that Mrs. S had about herself. On several occasions she voiced the following concern: "Who will I have to vent to after we stop meeting?" The therapist also had his own reservations about Mrs. S's ability to maintain her positive parenting practices without support. However, the therapist did appreciate and was able to point out to her the growing independence she had developed recently. Mrs. S and the therapist were able to note together her increased initiative with Barbara, as well as Barbara's greater ease in sharing her worries more directly with her mother. Once again, the opportunity to discuss these issues together seemed to provide the support that allowed Mrs. S to leave treatment with a fair degree of confidence to carry on on her own. In fact, during the last session, she was able to talk about her plan to turn more to her own adult friends in order to secure the support she would need.

Discussion

It was clear that because of the impact of the divorce on Mrs. S, she became less able to function as a parent. She had many reality stresses (income, education, adult relationships) as well as the internal stresses of severe loss, which led to feelings of fatigue and depression. The therapist took on the role of a nurturer and, within the relationship, provided a form of sustenance through interest, availability, and support. Therefore, I use the term "transference parenting" to describe this process. As with parent guidance, this is a supportive form of psychotherapy in which insight and understanding do not have a major role. The critical aspect is the parenting relationship that is experienced in the transference between the child's parent and the therapist.

BIBLIOGRAPHY

Arnold, E. (1978). *Helping Parents Help Their Children*. New York: Brunner/
Mazel.
Mishne, I. (1983). *Clinical Work with Children*. New York: Free Press.
Sandler, J., Kennedy, H., & Tyson, R. (1980). *The Technique of Child Psycho-
analysis: Discussions with Anna Freud*. Cambridge, MA: Harvard University
Press.
Weisberger, E. (1980). Concepts in ego psychology as applied to work with par-
ents. In: J. M. Mishne (Ed.), *Psychotherapy and Training in Clinical Social
Work*. New York: Gardner Press.

5

~

Treatment of
the Parent–Child Relationship

There are certainly situations in which the parent work needs to go beyond the technique of parent guidance. We are aware that in the advice–informational approach we do not deal with unconscious conflicts or unconscious unions between parents and child that often are a fundamental source of the difficulty. Do we then focus on the individual psychopathology of the parents and develop simultaneous treatments? It is also clear that a total treatment effort is often not absolutely necessary to help parents understand how their internal lives can impinge on their parenting role.

A number of authors have articulated a need for a variety of "in-between" techniques (between advice–guidance and total treatment) that would deal with some of the unconscious aspects of the parent–child relationship. Ackerman (1958), for example, noted that we should have a "hierarchy of levels of contact, categories of psychotherapeutic process differentiated in accordance with the depth of influence to be exerted on the personality of the parents" (p. 73). However, although he describes the "first level" as guidance or reeducation, and the reorganization of unconscious function as the

This chapter is reprinted, with changes, from "Treatment of Parent–Child Relationship," by M. Chethik, *Journal of the American Academy of Child Psychiatry*, Summer 1976, Vol. 15, No. 3, pp. 453–463. Copyright 1976 by Yale University Press. Reprinted by permission.

"deepest level," he says very little about the in-between grades. In fact, surprisingly, there are only a small number of papers that are relevant to or deal at all with these "in-between" areas of work (Levy, 1973; Cutter & Hallowitz, 1962; Slavson, 1952; Frailberg, 1954).

The purpose of this chapter is to articulate one mode of treatment in the middle range of work with parents, which I have chosen to call "treatment of the parent–child relationship." It is a process of ego clarification and *limited insight therapy* through which the unconscious meanings of a child for the parents can become evident. Despite the fact that interpretations and uncovering interventions are used, this process contains important boundaries that limit the transference and control transference regressions. In the course of the chapter, a number of case vignettes are presented, and a discussion of the principles that shape this technique follows.

The type of therapeutic management of parents described herein was a customary approach in the child psychiatric clinics of the 1950s and early 1960s. Caseworkers and the occasional psychiatrist working with parents had evolved an exploratory technique that was focused on the parent–child relationship but involved the various developmental and psychological factors within the parent that impinged on his or her relations with the child. The techniques were derived from the psychoanalytic orientation of the staff members, and, differing in several ways from psychoanalytic psychotherapy of the adult for his or her own emotional problems, they often brought about change in other areas of the parent's life beyond his or her capacities for parenting. Case studies reported during those years, in which the work of each member of the team was described, frequently suggest such approaches with the parent.

The last decade of mental health orientation emphasized a more reality-centered approach to parents, or family therapy if exploratory management was considered necessary. In many of the older child psychiatric facilities, what we refer to "as treatment of the parent–child relationship" undoubtedly continues, and staff members have adapted it to their private work. However, the more contemporary literature on child mental health does not provide examples of such work, nor is there much indication in the literature that casework or child psychiatric practitioners value it today.

The rationale of the approach is readily illustrated with the child case that reaches an impasse after a period of work, and we become aware that the momentum of treatment has stimulated some intense anxieties within a parent. When the parents are helped to understand and gain some perspective on what they are reliving through the child, the treatment process proceeds again. We do not immediately refer the parent for direct personal psychotherapy, and it is common practice to work these temporary impasses through. Typically, some modified interpretation is necessary, some sector psychotherapy is accomplished, and some unconscious fantasy is illuminated. Why do we lack a body of literature on a common and often needed practice? I can only conclude that this kind of work is unfortunately considered low-status and second-class psychotherapy: this form of treatment is not considered the "essential work," while the glamour lies in the articulation of the direct work with the child. I consider this pejorative aura and stigma particularly unfortunate because much skill, sensitivity, and subtle technique are often required to help a parent (as a parent) in a significant and fundamental way. And we are also fully aware that treatment with the child very often prospers or flounders depending on the work with the parent.

CLINICAL MATERIAL

Mark and His Mother

Mark was 6 years of age when he came to treatment because of a history of many behavior difficulties, particularly impulsive rage and outbursts, which were fully described in Chapter 1. Mark displayed a diffuse aggressiveness, a striking out that often appeared unprovoked. During treatment, his accompanying fantasies showed that Mark feared sadistic attack, and his aggression warded off imagined danger. Further, he often provoked because he longed to be physically controlled so that he could gratify intense passive aims.

It was clear from the history that a long-standing fighting relationship existed between mother and son. In the weekly meetings with the mother, Mrs. L was extremely cooperative and consciously and quickly (on advice) established more effective limits in the home, which helped to begin to control Mark's acting out. When we came to understand that some of Mark's chaos sprang from intense excitements, Mrs. L (on the home front) established privacy in the bathroom and curtailed Mark's visits to her bedroom when she dressed. She utilized parent guidance well.

After several months of treatment, a daredevil theme became prominent in Mark's behavior. In the office, he climbed extensively; it was as if he were challenged by an obstacle and sought to master it. For instance, it became important for him to determine whether he could climb to the high windowsill and sit there. But this danger was not enough. He waited to see whether he could move across the windowsill; when that was accomplished, he attempted to do it in a standing position, and on and on. Slowly, it became more evident that Mark's mother played an important part in this counterphobic method of handling danger.

In a session with the therapist, the mother related that Mark, a nonswimmer, had wandered off to the neighborhood pool. The family had been terribly worried for a number of hours, but as she related the frightening event, a characteristic smile of pure pleasure illuminated her face. Mark was fantastically resourceful: He had found the pool himself seven blocks from home; he had persuaded the guard that he could enter despite the rule mandating that he needed a parent and the fact that he was well under 48 inches, the minimum height of admission. (In his therapy at this point, Mark was preoccupied with fears of drowning). His mother related all such events, all difficult situations and narrow escapes that Mark was involved in, as high adventures and gave clear indications of an underlying intense pleasure. It was clear that a good deal of Mark's frightening chance taking was being libidinally reinforced by Mrs. L. She was aware and accepted that although Mark's escapades frightened her, they also provided a part of her with some pleasure. These reactions became an area of mutual work between mother and therapist.

Throughout the therapist's contacts with the mother, he was impressed by her special identification with Mark. Whereas Mark might be more disturbed than his two brothers, she pointed out, he also had unique potentialities. He was brighter than they were, he had a special tenacity the others did not have, and he was the most attractive child. She could always get the older brother, Jason, to do what she wanted; he would dress himself with the clothing she had laid out for him without question. But if Mark determined he wanted to wear something of his own choosing, she could stand on her head and it would make no difference. As she related these incidents, her characteristic smile conveyed her obvious pleasure at the manliness that Mark displayed.

Her special tie to Mark had started early. When he had been born, she had felt that he was particularly attractive, partly because he had been completely covered with hair. The family joke was that they would leave the hospital to go directly to the barbershop. In addition, when Mrs. L was a child, her own hairiness had been a family topic for years. She had been a happy child, she felt, but had always had a rough time with her mother.

In order to maintain herself, Mrs. L had had to fight her own mother every inch of the way. It was not that her mother was mean, she felt, but that she had always wanted to be the complete boss. Mrs. L recalled that when she was organizing a "sweet 16" party, her mother had tried to take over all the arrangements. When the daughter had reacted, her mother had continued to interfere, and the girl had moved the party to a friend's house where she could manage it completely by herself. This pattern of clear assertion had continued even during Mrs. L's married life. Her mother would wonder whether she was keeping the dishes in the "right" place; she had new suggestions for furniture arrangement, and so on. Mrs. L, of course, would totally resist all ideas, as a result of which mother and daughter highly respected each other. This mutual esteem was in contrast to the relationship between Mrs. L's mother and her younger sister, who acted like a child and was very dependent on her mother.

With this history, Mrs. L could respond to the therapist's interpretations that she cherished the feisty little Mark who would never be beaten down, as it recalled and expressed her own feisty struggles with her mother. Part of her, of course, knew that Mark needed firm and authoritative limits, but another part inside her wanted to see Mark never knuckle down or be crushed by the authorities around him. As Mrs. L became increasingly aware that her limit setting would not choke the spirit out of Mark, she could effectively take command with less and less ambivalence. She could also with skill anticipate when Mark's "manly" defiance would promote her own subtle pleasure, and she went far in mastering any inappropriate messages she had been conveying to Mark. She also worked on new areas in which Mark's tenacity and activity could be appropriately expressed.

Matthew and His Father

Matthew, a 10-year-old youngster in residential treatment who was diagnosed as a borderline psychotic child. He was tall and extremely thin, and immediately alienated the staff by his overdramatic, shrill, pseudo-affective way of relating. Most striking about Matthew was his highly developed fantasy life: Matthew played out in soliloquy, with great animation, cartoon characters who warded off all sorts of attacks. Although it was felt that the institution had a great deal to offer Matthew, there was concern about the parents, who seemed to have totally decathected their child. The therapist believed that little progress would ultimately be made unless the gulf between Matthew and his parents could be bridged. Part of the goal in the first year of work with the M family was to understand the nature of the impasse between father and son.

Mr. M was a self-employed accountant, a rather charming, urbane man who had strong passive–dependent longings. He complained a great deal about his work, worked long hours, felt as though he were on a treadmill, and felt completely drained by it. He thought he did poorly financially as compared with other accountants; he feared getting into debt by buying a lot of extra equipment, yet having the equipment would make him much more efficient. But he was not a risktaker in his business. He also felt that his secretary ran his office and made too many decisions, but he did not want to fire her: She had been with him for many years, it would be hard or impossible to replace her, and she made things run smoothly every day. After all, she knew all of his clients very well. When he came home from work, he had just enough energy to turn on the TV. He could do that for the major part of the weekend, but he worried that he was not keeping up with his professional reading. He was concerned he was falling behind professionally.

He slowly acknowledged that there was a chasm between him and his son. He felt enormous tension when he was with Matthew, and their weekend contacts exhausted him. When the therapist helped him articulate his concerns about Matthew (What specifically made him uneasy?), he complained about Matthew's artistic flavor. He felt Matthew had a strange way of talking; he sounded high and shrill. He seemed interested in music all the time and always overdramatized a story. Why was he so often in the company of girls on campus? He was concerned about how thin Matthew looked and that he was "built" very poorly. The therapist clarified with Mr. M that he was not only worried that Matthew was not an all-American boy, but he was really scared that Matthew was a "queer."

Mr. M expressed intense feeling that in some way he had been at fault. This had been a major worry he had been harboring. Had he been responsible for raising this kind of child? He himself did not pursue many activities traditionally regarded as manly: he did not like woodwork, he was not a camper; and he was not very much interested in cars. He noted that since he was small he had been interested in classical music. He had been a Mozart lover, and he recalled that as an adolescent he was upset when he learned through a historical biography that Mozart was a homosexual.

A major area of preoccupation was Mr. M's "maternal" role toward Matthew when Matthew was young. He was the person who had been able to soothe and calm Matthew, not his wife, and Mr. M expressed a great deal of rage at his wife for having forced him into that position. Now he realized he was frightened of the effects of his handling: Had he kept Matthew on his lap too often, had he tried to compensate for his wife? He knew that he had suddenly withdrawn from

Matthew a number of years ago, and he retrospectively understood that much of his uneasiness came from his fear of the boy's femininity.

As this material emerged, Mr. M's anxiety could be clarified. The therapist then also had an opportunity to delineate clearly Matthew's problems. Matthew did not struggle fundamentally with his sexual identity: He was concerned about having an identity at all. The therapist could discuss with Mr. M Matthew's fears that the real world would not provide pleasure and Matthew's primitive fears that the world would destroy him. It was because of these fears that Matthew sought the company of little girls, because he projected his fears of intense aggressive attack by the boys; and his theatrical pseudo-affect defended him against real interpersonal relationships that he feared so much.

As Mr. M gained a sense of relief that he had not unalterably damaged his son, he relaxed with Matthew. They began to play ball together and went bowling. Matthew learned from his father how to use the family lawn mower under supervision, and he began to accompany his father to his accounting office for the first time.

Matthew and His Mother

Matthew's mother hated the institution. The staff handled Matthew poorly, she said. He was dressed badly, his bureau and room were a mess, food was poorly served, and the program allowed youngsters endless free time without adequate supervision. As Mrs. M complained and found little virtue in the treatment effort, the therapist sensed that she was attacking the institution and its staff to ward off their anticipated criticism. As she spoke of life with Matthew during the early years, it was clear that *he* had been impossible. He had never allowed himself to be comforted and had cried all of his waking hours—only the vibrations of a car ride calmed him momentarily. When he began to make sounds, *he* had chattered incessantly and spoke nonsense without letup. When he had begun to walk and toddle about, *he* had tolerated no limits and had embarrassed her constantly at the supermarket and on the street. He had been like a rope around her neck, an albatross. During those years, she had "hated" him, had felt imprisoned within the home, and she acknowledged that some of those feelings might even find their way into the mother–child relationship at present. Once in a great while in therapeutic work, there was a crack in Mrs. M's armor. For example, as she showed Matthew's baby book, she commented gently how Matthew had resembled her physically as a child, and she caressed and patted a lock of his hair that had been saved from his first year of life. But these moments were rare.

During one session she was vehement in her condemnation of Ed, one of the most effective child care staff members, who had developed a fine relationship with Matthew. Ed, she felt, coddled Matthew. When it was time for lunch and Matthew isolated himself in his room, Ed spoke to him softly about leaving his room. Didn't they have rules in the cottage? Why was Matthew an exception? Matthew was quickly learning how to manipulate Ed, as he would the entire staff. On this occasion, and many subsequent ones, the therapist interpreted that Mrs. M had very mixed feelings about Ed: Part of her wished she could handle her son as gently and effectively as Ed. Yet it was hard for her, because she was very frightened of the soft feelings within her.

For a period of time, Mrs. M spoke of her present aversions to Matthew on his infrequent home visits. Matthew was shadowing her, and she had to get away. Why was he always in the kitchen when she was cooking? She described how she planned meticulously for every hour of the weekend. Again, it was noted that perhaps she adopted the role of "manager" because she was frightened of the role of mother. On this occasion, she began to weep. She told the therapist for the first time that she was waking up at night repeatedly: Her images were of Matthew at the cottage, sad, alone, and totally cut off from the world.

This material ushered in a period of intense mourning. She had always felt she had lost her chance with her son. She described how she could never reach him, how terrible she had felt when he turned to his father every time he had fallen down and injured himself. Time and time again she saw the multiple ways he clearly showed an aversion to her. Mrs. M cried constantly for a period of time as soon as she crossed the threshold in the therapist's office, and it was clear that she was reacting to the lost opportunity to be a mother to her young son.

Slowly, her images of Matthew then changed and softened. He was no longer only manipulative: She knew when he was frightened and sad, and she recognized the defenses of anger and withdrawal within him. She became effectively empathic with Matthew, and her relationship to the staff became much more cooperative.

DISCUSSION

What are the criteria, principles, and particular problems that are inherent in this specific parent–child focus?

There are a number of criteria that should be considered before utilizing the techniques employed in these cases. In general, parents who can make effective use of this process have a level of ego intactness and psychological-mindedness that make them accessible to limited insight therapy. In the preceding situations, it was felt that the parents could clearly identify with the particular goals of this treatment effort. The M family came to recognize that there was a great distance between themselves and Matthew, and Mrs. L was concerned about the messages she had been delivering to her son Mark despite herself. In this work, there was a period during which the problematic aspects of the parent–child relationship became ego-alien to these parents, and there was a conscious resolution to modify them. Therefore, these parents had the capacity for some effective self-observation. An implicit therapeutic alliance was formed: The therapist would help them understand the nature of these impasses with their children and of the roles they had played.

This particular approach, although it is child-focused, provides opportunity to deal with some of the appropriate criticisms coming from the family literature. We have read a great deal about the dangers of accepting the child as the identified patient. It is often noted that parents mask their family, marital, and individual problems by making the child the conscious repository of all of the pathology. Much of the aim of this technique is indeed to deal with the interactive and mutually pathological interplays within the family. After a period of time, it was seen that Mark was not alone in the L family with his pathology; his need to function as the fearless daredevil had been constantly libidinally reinforced by his mother. Within the M family, Matthew could not enter the real world unless he felt there were ties to, and gratification coming from, his primary objects.

Within the scope of this technique, one can carefully evaluate the parents' need to externalize their impact on their child. There are considerable advantages in being able slowly to include the family and to clarify their roles in the child's pathology. Often, parents need the defense of the "bad" or "sick child," and with the aforementioned techniques, a therapist can titrate the amount of confrontation and clarification of parental contribution. It was clear that Mrs. L and Mr. M could quickly come to acknowledge that they were involved. But Mrs. M needed to attack and criticize the agency for a long period of time until she had established a trusting relationship and felt there would be no retaliation.

We are often too quick to conclude that a parental request that asks us to remain focused on the child smacks of defensiveness and denial. The parents may be providing us with another implicit request, namely, to help them function as effective parents, as emotional educators, and as teachers, and this request emerges appropriately from the impetus of the phase of parenthood in which they are. I have found that many parents have seized on the opportunity of some form of parent–child work because of a healthy and appropriate guilt that they carry. They are aware internally that they have contributed to the present problem. This form of treatment speaks to their parenting need, for it provides an opportunity to clarify, undo, and reverse some of the past mishandling. For example, there was much that Mr. M wanted to teach Matthew, and his effort in therapy was to understand directly those aspects of himself that had made it impossible for him to relate to his son.

What problems emerge in a limited insight therapy? Often, in this process, unconscious material is elicited and can then be interpreted. Mrs. L had had no awareness that she was identified with Mark's rebelliousness and was reliving her own childhood struggles with her mother. Mr. M, although intensely aware of his uneasiness with his son, learned through his own therapeutic work that Matthew represented his feared and projected femininity. Mrs. M came to understand that her rage with her son embodied her failure as a mother and woman generally and that she was simultaneously terrified of her softness.

Not only is the therapy a process of insight development, but there are obvious reconstructions. These parents have learned that their inappropriate affect responses (rage, withdrawal) to their children are not reality based but come from earlier childhood contexts (repetition of their struggles with their parents, or internal struggles with parts of themselves). In fact, creating and reliving within a historical context was enormously helpful in removing the child as the target and source of the family pathology. Yet I have found that despite the intense process of self-observation work with memories, affects, and dream material, transference and regressions are limited and controlled. This occurs because there are constant opportunities to redefine the boundaries of the work. With all parents, there is a constant question—how has this material (e.g., the struggle you had with your mother) influenced what goes on between you and your child now? These comments immediately address their current parenting image and move them from the angry, frightened child role they had assumed during the treatment hour.

This technique is explicitly a form of sector psychotherapy

(Deutsch & Murphy, 1954–1955) with delineated goals that particularly meet the developmental needs of children. We are aware that in order to minimize pathology, we need to intervene early, as close to the developmental interference as possible. Often, even effective individual personal psychotherapy of a parent comes too late, because even though he or she may make significant gains over the years, the child is beyond many of the significant developmental stages. Treatment of the parent–child relationship as a technique aims to focus immediately on the interlocking struggle between parent and child so that fixations will not become entrenched and constantly reinforced.

BIBLIOGRAPHY

Ackerman, N. (1958). *Psychodynamics of Family Life*. New York: Basic Books.

Cutter, A., & Hallowitz, D. (1962). Different approaches to treatment of the child and the parents. *American Journal of Orthopsychiatry* 22:15–159.

Deutsch, F., & Murphy, W. F. (1954–1955). *The Clinical Interview*. New York: International Universities Press.

Fraiberg, S. (1954). Counseling for the parents of the very young child. *Social Casework* 35:47–57.

Kessler, J. (1966). *Psychopathology of Childhood*. Englewood Cliffs, NJ: Prentice-Hall.

Levy, D. M. (1973). Attitude therapy. *American Journal of Orthopsychiatry* 7:103–113.

Slavson, S. (1952). *Child Psychotherapy*. New York: Columbia University Press.

III

~

The Process
of Treatment:
The Fundamentals

Introduction

This part focuses on some of the fundamental information that the practitioner needs in order to manage and set goals for a patient's psychotherapy. The therapist needs to understand how the child's *pathology* will shape the treatment techniques, and to understand the basic *psychotherapeutic concepts* that will help him or her organize the treatment effort.

THE PSYCHOPATHOLOGIES

This part introduces the reader to both the major psychopathologies of childhood as well as to the specific treatment process for each of these pathologies. There is a chapter on the neurotic child (Chapter 6), as well as chapters on children with character pathology (Chapter 7) and borderline and narcissistic disturbances (Chapters 8 and 9). This part concludes with a chapter (Chapter 10) on reactive disorders in children, illustrated by the treatment of children in divorce and bereavement.

Throughout these chapters the general natures of the various pathologies are discussed. From this material, for example, the reader can come to understand what is meant by childhood neurosis and how it differs from character pathology in children. In each chapter, in addition to a general discussion of the pathology, there is a full case illustration and a discussion of the underlying psychodynamics.

Each disturbance presents the therapist with different treatment problems and calls for different techniques and interventions. The major focus of each chapter highlights these issues. Here I describe the process of insight-oriented psychotherapy with neurotic children, the process of defense analysis with children with character pathology, the supportive techniques employed with severely disturbed borderline youngsters, and other therapeutic approaches.

THE PSYCHOTHERAPEUTIC CONCEPTS

An additional theme weaves through this part of the book as well. In the literature there are a number of basic concepts of psychotherapy that help the practitioner to organize and evaluate the ongoing process of treatment. These concepts have been derived primarily from adult psychodynamic psychotherapy, and I will define them and reshape these ideas in child terms. They may be outlined in the following way:

The Therapeutic Alliance
Resistance
Transference
Interventions

The Therapeutic Alliance

The therapeutic alliance is defined as the nontransference part of the relationship between patient and therapist. It is the reasonable rapport that the patient has with the therapist that enables the patient to work purposefully in the treatment and share the goals of the treatment. An earlier example of an emerging therapeutic alliance is described in Chapter 1. It occurred with the patient Mark, when he became reflective well into the treatment. He told the therapist it was very hard for him to be good. He began a series of confessions about Gary (not Mark) who was wild but afraid of ghosts, frightened by robbers, and Gary even made "doo" in his pants. The therapeutic alliance is the observing part of the relationship rather than the experiencing part (Greenson, 1967; Sandler, Holder, & Dare, 1973). Contributions to the alliance are made by the patient, the therapist, and the structure of the treatment.

The patient implicitly makes many contributions in order to produce an effective alliance. He needs to be willing to produce material, to regress through fantasy or play, and to convey the nature of the regression to the therapist. An alliance implies some ability to use and mull over what the therapist observes. It also implies some motivation of the patient to overcome his illness. For an effective alliance, the patient must have some capacity to tolerate the frustration of therapy (e.g., when the therapist comments on painful issues or points out problematic behaviors).

These capacities are based, in part, on the quality of earlier object relationships, particularly the capacity for "basic trust" (Erikson, 1963). They are based also on the development of particular ego functions, including memory, intelligence, verbal capacity, and the capacity for self-observation. The child patient has a limited ability to think about himself, and he typically finds it painful to feel that there are "worries" and problems. The alliance with the child becomes an "immature therapeutic alliance," which depends on the positive relationship with the therapist rather than a sharing of common goals.

The therapist contributes to the alliance in a number of ways. Above all, the therapist implicitly conveys that he or she wants to help the patient become well. He or she does this through the persistent pursuit of uncomfortable material, the capacity to produce insight, and continuous work with resistances, all within a context of a caring demeanor. For example, in Chapter 1, in the early work with Mark there was a period when the child was terrified and out of control. The therapist worked to produce a safe surround, as the blocks flew and the chairs were overturned. Mark was not rejected, and slowly he contained his actions. The therapist became a safe and dependable affect regulator, which contributed to the alliance the two gradually developed. Another important aspect of the therpist's contribution is his or her neutrality. The therapist need not impose his or her own standards and values.

The structure of the sessions also contributes to the development of the alliance. The fact that there is a fixed quality to the session, that there are regular and orderly working routines, that the therapist conveys that the hour is important (through rarely missing a session, making few schedule changes, and not allowing interruptions), all contribute to a sense of security and enhance the alliance. The therapist strives to create a work environment that supports the unfolding of the child's inner world. In work with children, the fixed quality of the hour is more commonly interfered with than in adult work. For example, the accompanying parent may, at times, seek to talk with the therapist before he or she sees the child, therefore encroaching on the child's treatment hour. Although one cannot always reject out-of-hand this request, asking whether it can wait until after the patient's hour conveys therapist's regard for the importance of the child patient's working time.

As noted earlier, an *immature alliance* is based on the child's positive relationship with the adult therapist. The adult becomes trusted as a helping person, a person whose lead is followed, and the child therefore becomes more willing to work. This was quite evident in the work with Douglas (Chapter 3). After a period of Douglas's fearing the therapist as the dreaded attacker, we saw signs of a growing positive attachment. As the relationship grew, Douglas's destructive actions turned to vigorous play—Jack the Ripper—and his affection for the "worry doctor" became evident as Douglas found a new way to play out his intense fears. A major aspect of the immature alliance is the positive attachment (Sandler, Kennedy, & Tyson, 1980). This is often based on a libidinal component—a love relationship founded on earlier aspects of the positive relationship between parent and child.

In child work, an alliance with the child alone is not enough. One of the functions of the child therapist is to develop an effective alliance with the family (Sandler, Holder, & Dare, 1973). Just as the child needs the parent's approval of a playmate, activity, or toy, the child must come to feel that the parent approves of the psychotherapist and the therapy.

Resistance

Generally, resistance is defined as those forces that perpetuate the status quo of the neurosis (illness). Resistance operates against the reasonable ego and the wish to change. It interferes with the ability to remember, gain, and assimilate insight (Greenson, 1967; Langs, 1973; Sandler, Holder, & Dare, 1973). Resistances may be conscious, preconscious, and/or unconscious.

A major part of every treatment is dealing with the phenomenon of resistance, which accompanies the course of treatment each step of the way. Therefore, the most cooperative patient will simultaneously evidence resistance, inasmuch as it is natural for all human beings to repress pain and shameful memories, experiences, and affects. For example, even when a patient is bringing forth a dream, the therapist meets resistance as the dream material is a disguised version of some unconscious idea.

When resistance is used colloquially, therapists often comment about the "resistant patient," thinking of someone who is overtly noncooperative or missing sessions. This use of the term "resistance" is often applied to children more generally, because they overtly take flight from treatment, make evident their wishes to leave, or deny the entire process. Technically, however, this is only a form of conscious resistance, and all patients manifest many forms of resistance.

The therapist's internal response to resistance is that it interferes with the treatment. Actually, the mode of resistance often informs the therapist. The reason is that the process by which a patient resists illuminates how the patient's ego is working. It is the ego of the patient that has developed many mechanisms to keep intolerable issues hidden from consciousness. Thus, in helping a patient understand and verbalize his resistances, the therapist helps the patient to gain insight into how a major part of his personality operates. It is not unusual that the understanding of the defenses the patient employs may be the most crucial part of the treatment. For example, after a period of work in the case of Mark (Chapter 1), he became self-observant about his "lion feelings" and how they emerged when he was scared. The therapist had done a great deal of work on his defense/resistance of "passive to active." Although Mark did not know exactly what frightened him, he gradually became sensitive to the emergence of these feelings, and this led him to the ability to contain this acting out (lion feelings).

A number of authors enumerate many classes of resistances (Sandler, Holder, & Dare, 1973). It is helpful to conceptualize three major categories of resistance: (1) ego resistances—the prevalent defensive processes of the patient as they emerge in treatment; (2) id resistance—particular instinctual activities that are used to ward off insight (for example, a patient who fears underlying homosexual wishes acts continuously to prove his heterosexual prowess, denying his homosexuality); (3) superego resistances—resistances linked to unconscious guilt and the need for punishment. The conscience of the patient works against the treatment, inasmuch as progress with his or her illness would be experienced as too great a reward. Generally, id and superego resistances are more formidable to work through than ego resistances.

Transference

A very important aspect of the psychotherapy experience is the phenomenon of transference. Transference is defined as the patient's experience of feelings, drives, attitudes, fantasies, and defenses toward a person in the present that do not fit that person but are a repetition of reactions originating in regard to significant persons of early childhood, unconsciously displaced onto figures of the present (Greenson, 1967). A present figure can be anyone significant in the person's current life. Thus, Douglas (Chapter 3) feared the attacking worry doctor because he "transferred" the feelings he had about his father onto this new man in his life. With the regressive pull of the process of psychotherapy, the therapist will often take on various transference roles.

When the phenomenon of transference occurs within the therapy, attempting to understand and clarify the distorted transference can be either of irreplaceable value to the patient or a major threat to the treatment. The patient is living out and reenacting the past, with the immediate and intense feelings of the present. On one hand, this can be the key to many insights, and because of the quality of the affective experience, it can often provide the patient with a sense of conviction regarding the origin of the events. However, often when the patient begins to experience these affects toward the therapist, this can stir up powerful resistances that can prove to be major obstacles to any further work.

There is a variety of transference in child work: (1) character transference, (2) transference of past relationships, (3) transference of current relationships, and (4) the therapist as an object of externalization.

Character transference is a *habitual* mode of relating to classes of people that is inappropriate to those people but emerges from significant past experiences. Both Mark (Chapter 1) and Douglas (Chapter 3) immediately related to adults (authority) with characteristic fear and a subsequent defensive "tough guy" stance. They habitually reacted to new adults as though they were the attacking fathers.

Transference of past relationships refers to derivatives of meaningful and significant relationships of the past that emerge from the treatment situation after a period of psychotherapeutic work, Again, they are inappropriate reactions to the therapist. The past experience is repressed, but the effects of the experience produce current disturbances in the form of symptoms or troubling behaviors. The process of therapy helps to revive the wishes, fears, and unconscious memories associated with these past experiences through the living relationship with the therapist. This differs from character transference, which is global, expressed with many people, and usually evident at the start of treatment. The transference of past relationships emerges slowly in the course of treatment under the pressure of repetition compulsion.

Another major source of transference is the displacement of current internal issues between the child and family members onto the therapist. This phenomenon is called *transference of current relationships*. The child patient often expresses forbidden affects he has toward parents or siblings in the treatment hour, as the therapy situation feels safer. There are two major sources of these displacements: reality conflicts stemming from current family issues and developmental conflicts that are appropriate to the age level of the child.

The last general type of transference is the inappropriate use of the *therapist as an object of externalization*. In this process, the child splits off and displaces one aspect of an internal conflict onto the therapist and thereby experiences some relief. For example, consider a typical process in adolescence. Many teenagers experience intense sexual impulses, and rather than struggle internally (e.g. "I shouldn't live out these feelings"), they externalize the control pressures (superego components of the conflict), displacing them onto parents or other authorities. They repress their own guilt and instead see parents as imposing a "guilt trip" on them. During treatment, patients use this form of splitting their internal conflicts, attributing the uncomfortable aspects to the therapist.

Interventions

Interventions are techniques (usually verbal) used by the therapist to ameliorate the problems of the patient. In psychodynamic psychotherapy with neurotic patients, these techniques are typically uncovering processes (to "uncover" the warded-off internal life) whose purpose is to provide insight to the patient (Langs, 1973). The process is often conceived in four steps:

1. *Confrontation*, wherein the phenomenon in question is made evident and explicit to the patient's ego.
2. *Clarification*, during which the phenomenon is sharpened and further clarified (blends with process of confrontation).
3. *Interpretion*, the process of making the unconscious meaning of the phenomenon conscious to the patient. This may include simply providing the meaning of the phenomenon, but also may include the source, the historical context connected to the phenomenon.
4. *Working through*, processes after an interpretation is given and some insight is gained. This may include repetitions and elaborated explorations of the meaning of the insight, assessing the resistance or symptoms connected with it, and seeing its effect on daily living in current relationships.

The confrontation and clarification aspects are critical parts of the intervention process, because the patient must slowly become prepared for an interpretation. Only when a patient accepts and observes some aspect of his own functioning, and finds it somewhat ego-alien, can an interpretation be useful. The interpretation is clearly the heart of the intervention process—the process of making some unconscious aspect of the patient conscious—and it provides the opportunity for insight and potential for change.

There is no formula for effective timing for an interpretation. Intuitively, a therapist learns about the patient's capacity to hear, and this capacity provides clues about what, when, and how to interpret. The internal state of the therapist will affect his or her sense of timing. Beginning therapists often want to share their insights and discoveries immediately, because they seek affirmation of their effectiveness. New therapists may also be frightened about producing pain and disturbing the young patient, and therefore may withhold necessary confrontations and interpretations.

A sense of this process is described in the work with Mark. It took quite a few months before Mark could accept the therapist's idea that he had "lion feelings." The therapist was using confrontation and clarification to bring Mark's acting-out behavior into sharp focus as something they could think about together. At times the therapist noted that Mark's lion feelings were so strong that they even surprised Mark (e.g., Mark broke things he cared about or became a daredevil). These interventions touched on behavior that

Mark was aware of—he had a conscious or preconscious idea that he had a "fighting problem." When the lion feelings became something that was familiar in the hour, the therapist could go further. What made these lion feelings errupt? The therapist noted that when Mark became scared, he needed to push the scary feelings away. At that point the therapist made an interpretation. Mark was totally unaware of the motivation of his tough guy, fighting behavior. With these interpretations and Mark's new wish to control himself, the therapist was free to explore many things that made Mark (and all boys) scared.

These psychotherapeutic concepts that I have defined will repeatedly emerge in the body of the forthcoming cases. I will illustrate how they emerge, how they will help organize the therapist's thinking, and how understanding them leads to effective interventions.

BIBLIOGRAPHY

Greenson, R. (1967). *The Techniques and Practice of Psychoanalysis*. New York: International Universities Press.

Langs, R. (1973). *The Technique of Psychoanalytic Psychotherapy*. New York: Jason Aronson.

Sandler, J., Holder A., & Dare, C. (1973). *The Patient and the Analyst*. New York: International Universities Press.

Sandler, J., Kennedy, H., & Tyson, R. (1980). *The Technique of Child Analysis: Discussion with Anna Freud*. Cambridge, MA: Harvard University Press.

6

~

Treatment of
the Neurotic Child

This chapter has a twofold purpose. A major focus is on the process of treating neurotic children—that is, specific techniques highlighting the use of uncovering interpretations and the utilization of transference are presented. Another purpose is further discussion and illustration of the use of the relevant psychotherapeutic concepts. Both the concepts themselves and the techniques used with the neurotic child are discussed in conjunction with a clinical presentation.

The case of Fred, an 11-year-old obsessional youngster in residential placement is presented, and a technical assessment follows the evaluative material. Fred presents somewhat like an adult patient for two reasons. First, he is an obsessional patient. Obsessional children often precociously develop many ego functions (e.g., memory, intelligence, secondary thought processes) and are therefore able to develop highly structured and enduring defenses that have an adult-like form (there is a stabilization of their egos, and they tend to use verbalization extensively). Second, Fred is moving out of childhood into early adolescence, and we see the natural development of many ego functions. Thus, when psychotherapeutic concepts are discussed

A version of this chapter, "The Therapy of an Obsessive Compulsive," by M. Chethik, was published in *Journal of the American Academy of Child Psychiatry*, July 1969, Vol. 8, No. 3, pp. 465–484.

and illustrated in this chapter, there is something of an adult quality to the definitions.

FRED: BACKGROUND, HISTORY, AND THE PRESENTING PICTURE IN TREATMENT

Fred was in treatment for a 3-year period, between the ages of 11 and 14. During his treatment he lived at Sagebrook, a residential treatment center for emotionally disturbed children.

Fred had initially been referred because of growing problems during his latency years. His school performance had caused his parents increasing concern. Although he was well behaved and intelligent, he evidenced many severe symptoms that made it hard for him to function on a daily basis.

Within his home there had always been a great deal of tension. There was constant conflict between the parents. The mother complained of her husband's violence and uncontrollable rage with the children, his social bluntness and inappropriateness, and his "obsession" with dirt in the house (particularly in the bathroom). In turn, the husband felt that his wife was stubborn and insensitive to his needs and feelings. Both were aware of their marital difficulties.

The father was a driving, aggressive, successful businessman who tyrannized the household. In contrast, the mother was quiet and ineffective with her children. She lacked any self-assurance, and her constant self-questioning and self-effacing made it difficult for her to act decisively and set limits for her four children. The home was characterized by uproar during the day, with mother at the helm, and severe repression during the evening when father returned from work.

An evident fighting and sadistic interplay existed between father and son. Conflict between them had begun during Fred's earliest years. A pattern of stubborn refusal and resistance by Fred was met by overwhelming force and suppression by his father. During Fred's second year, he developed what his parents perceived to be some eating difficulties. He refused many foods, and the mother's anxiety and helplessness mounted. His father resolved to "make" Fred eat, and he was tied to the highchair for all evening meals. Similarly, it was the father who struggled with Fred about bowel training. Fred was often hit for his infractions, as this symptom particularly disturbed his father. Furthermore, the father handled Fred's insistence on climbing out of the crib by locking him in his room. During Fred's later childhood years, many little attempts at assertion were often similarly interpreted as "defiance." Coming in late for supper, climbing trees, and wading in a nearby brook were all events that were met with harsh and unrealistic punishments.

It is important to note that behind the father's "tough" appearance, there were glimpses of softness and fearfulness. As he described moments when his rage made him beat Fred, he became tearfully guilty and frightened by his own aggression. There were many occasions when he sought to undo the damage, and there were short-lived periods when father and son enjoyed each other.

Fred's own temper, however, became a dominant theme during his preschool and early elementary school years. The excessive roughness he exhibited with other children in nursery school at ages 3 and 4 had precipitated the initial contact with a guidance clinic. The clinic's impression was that Fred was a very tense and frightened child, as well as an enraged one. When Fred was 5½, his mother returned to the clinic because of Fred's continued impulsive aggression toward schoolmates and her difficulties in managing him at home. The mother also noted that although they did not get along well when they were together, Fred had many fears regarding separation from her, particularly in accepting baby-sitters.

During Fred's eighth year, his parents noted some important changes. Fred appeared much more polite and well behaved outside the home, but his academic problems and difficulties in going to sleep became acute. He was unable to concentrate, follow directions, or complete assignments. He developed fears of dirt, touching the walls, and going outside into the street. These fears could become severe and incapacitating. An extensive evaluation indicated that there were many internalized problems, and because there were multiple pressures within the home as well, placement was recommended. It took several years and increasing symptom intensity before placement was actually effected.

During Fred's initial year at Sagebrook, the effective outer controls that were developing were maintained. He still appeared to be a manageable youngster who was cooperative, conforming, and thoughtful.

From his first session, Fred seemed to take his treatment seriously. When he entered the room, he carefully laid down his jacket, seated himself at the edge of the chair facing the therapist, and stiffly proceeded to talk. Fred impressed the therapist as a "little intellectual." He was small and dark with a thin frame. His glasses appeared very prominent on his face, and his use of words and phrases indicated that he was well read and knowledgeable. Fred totally related to the treatment in this studious manner. He was intent on talking, and in the first year, with no exception, he never left the chair that faced the therapist for any reason (to use play equipment, go to the bathroom, or even stretch).

In the first session Fred outlined many difficulties and "deep worries" in abundant and precise detail, and although he spoke quietly and carefully, it was evident that he was quite pained and troubled about his symptoms.

He was worried about his schoolwork. He felt that he was slower in math than the other children. In the time that they were able to do four to five pages of a long division assignment, he would linger over one page. This was because he was concerned about errors, and he laboriously checked and rechecked his work. He felt that reading was a problem too. For some reason he needed to read very quickly. He read almost continuously and devoured many books weekly, but he was troubled because by rushing through the pages, he often did not have time to understand the content. He was interested in reading *sets* of books and was now working his way through a 25-volume series by the same publisher. (These books also had similar bindings.)

Fred mentioned some of his fears during that first hour, primarily fear of animals, and he elaborated on them during the first few weeks of treatment. He was concerned about bee stings and about the cats that came onto the campus. At night his imagination would sometimes control his thoughts, and the alley cats would turn into "bobcats" hiding behind the shade in his room. Mosquitoes became troubling, particularly because they extract blood; he described a fantasy of swallowing a mosquito while he was asleep. He feared the mosquito would find its way into his heart and pierce the wall with its stinger. He commented on the fantasy's irrationality, yet he noted he could not stop the growth of such worries. Sometimes in the morning he was convinced there was a bull under his bed. Afraid to put his feet on the floor because it would attract the animal, he would gather his clothing very quickly and dress in the bathroom. At times he would decide to lie quietly, but the elaboration and escalation of his fears would continue. The thought would come that as he lay still, the horns of the bull would soon pierce the mattress. Often one could sense in Fred the new underlying wishes and impulses breaking through, followed by the new elaborate fear–defense.

He was concerned about his eating habits. At times he ate little. Smells disturbed him, and the milk seemed to have a trace of ketchup. Pudding often had lumps in it, liver and tomatoes gave him a choking feeling, hamburgers had grease on them, and on and on. He often felt great disgust in the dining room. As with his animal fears, his food aversion would dramatically spread. Some days, only the long-established dislikes were avoided, but on other days, Fred might eat absolutely nothing at mealtimes. He vacillated. At times this was an external problem because of what he perceived as the horrible food standards at Sagebrook. At other times, however, he recognized that his eating difficulties existed at home and in restaurants as well. On one occasion during that early period he said, "If I didn't have to eat in order to live, I would give up food entirely."

There was also one plaguing memory. Fred wanted to confess that about a year prior to his placement, he threw a large rock and killed a baby mouse near his home. It left a red stain on the driveway. He had tried twice to wash the spot away, but for a month he had to walk by and see it every day. As he described his memory (which he repeatedly referred to), he could not contain the smile of pleasure that broke through. At the start of treatment, this memory was the only direct allusion to some problem with his inner aggression.

The therapist was somewhat surprised with these initial interviews. Surprised because they seemed so clearly to fit the well-defined structure of the obsessive–compulsive: the compulsive systems themselves, the doubting, the escalation and spread of fears, the intact, cold, sadistic memories, and so forth.

PSYCHODYNAMIC TECHNICAL ASSESSMENT

The purpose of the assessment was to understand and give meaning to the problematic behavior and/or symptoms that Fred evidenced. Fred appeared quite paralyzed in school, checking and rechecking his work. He was controlled by rituals or systems he had to live by. He *had* to read the books in order, or something terrible would happen. He was often frightened of going into the street, fearing attacks of animals. He showed a number of phobias. At times, he had problems eating because he was disgusted by the smells and the "lumps" in the food. There was also generalized guilt, as he thought about the plaguing memory of killing the baby mouse, or feared the attacks of the bobcats from the woods (form of punishment).

I. Drive Assessment

The clinical material highlighted that the major ongoing problem that Fred had was a struggle with his *aggressive drive*, focusing particularly on the *anal components* of that drive. History indicated that during Fred's early years (second and third years of life) he had been treated very severely by his father. Battles occurred around eating, toilet training, and issues of anatomy. This interplay appeared to have stimulated counteractive rage within Fred (pre-oedipal rage, as this occurred during that phase of development). In Fred's history there was evidence of his impulsivity as a child, but during latency and early adolescence, his aggression was highly defended against. Actually, he was seen as a youngster with an absence of aggression but one who was highly symptomatic.

The anal form of the aggressive drive is expressed in cruel and sadistic wishes, in desires to be messy and dirty. These components were not directly evident at all, but intensely warded off (defended against). Evidence of dirty, messy wishes were expressed in the opposite—Fred was disgusted by the "smells," the "lumpiness," and the textures of the food. Although Fred gave no evidence of his own sadism or cruelty, he feared the attacks of vicious, cruel animals in the environment (these specific defenses are discussed in the section on Ego Assessment). This sadism and messiness (anal forms of aggression) were salient issues for Fred, although in his perception they came from outside and not from within.

There were also some problems of *aggression* that seemed derived from the *phallic–oedipal period of development*. Normally, the aggressive drive in this phase of development is expressed in competition. Boys seek to be powerful men and pit themselves against other children and their fathers. Again in the history, the father had treated Fred very harshly when he had expressed his early manliness and prowess (climbing trees, exploring, etc.). Fred's difficulties in school appeared to be related to his problems in competition. The sense of power that youngsters express physically in early childhood is typically also expressed intellectually when they enter school. They compete by seeing who is the smartest and the quickest. Despite the fact that Fred was endowed with considerable intellectual gifts, he was unable to use them competitively and achievement was considerably impaired.

With respect to the *libidinal* nature of Fred's drives, the evaluation process provided relatively little material. One theme appeared to be Fred's penetration worries. He feared the piercing of the bull's horn and the mosquito sting. There had been a strong sado-masochistic interplay between father and son, and this kind of early interaction can promote a sense of passivity and excitement (anticipating attack), as well as the fears and rage already discussed. This suggests that one libidinal legacy could be translated into some homosexual wishes where Fred would fear/wish to be the penetrated female partner.

II. Ego Assessment

Generally, Fred's major ego functions appeared to be intact, and he seemed well endowed. He was highly intelligent, his memory functioned well, and his speech and vocabulary were extremely well developed. He was able to abstract well and had no problems with reality testing (distinguishing between an internal thought and an external reality). For example, when he became fearful of the "bob-cats" in the Sagebrook woods, he was aware that this fear was a product of his imagination and not a current reality.

Fred's ego was under a great deal of strain, and there were breakthroughs of anxiety (the indirect fears) when his defenses did not work adequately. This experience of anxiety was the basis for the subjective pain that Fred described during his first few sessions. His defenses were used primarily to ward off his experiencing his aggressive impulses consciously. The following are the defenses he used prominently:

1. *Isolation/intellectualization.* This process involves separating appropriate affects from actual events. Fred had a meticulous and detailed way of explaining all sorts of experiences, but he would not let himself experience the feeling components attached to these experiences. This was a method of warding off aggressive feelings.

2. *Undoing.* Undoing involves a need to perform some particular act to avoid a feeling of anxiety. Often the act is the opposite, or an "undoing," of a previous act. There is often a compulsive need to "undo." Fred evidenced many problems in school, and the mechanism of undoing was involved in his paralysis with his work. For example, he described being unable to do his math, and he needed to erase and recheck, erase and recheck his answers. Internally (uncon-

sciously), Fred was frightened that any actions (in this case, answering a question) were a sign of his aggression. He was frightened that any action could be a "mistake" (which in his mind was equated with a sadistic act), and he undid it by erasing and rechecking his work over and over again.

3. *Reaction formation.* With reaction formation, impulses are changed into their opposite; this mechanism is often associated with undoing. Fred was *repelled* and disgusted by the "smell" and the "lumpiness" of his food. Internally, the anal child finds enormous pleasure in dirt, and these impulses appeared to be intensely defended against by Fred. In addition, his sense of fairness and concern for others in his early period at Sagebrook, which seemed to be excessive, pushed away his internal wishes to hurt others. In general, this internally angry youngster was consciously good and compliant, orderly, and well mannered.

4. *Projection.* In this mechanism, the ego alters the source of the dangerous impulse from within and attributes it to someone (or something) else. The animals at Sagebrook carried the dangerous hurting impulses that were originally within Fred. They, rather than Fred, expressed the biting, attacking feelings.

5. *Displacement.* This mechanism also involves a shifting of the source of frightening perceptions but does not involve impulses from within. Fred was terrified of the rage of his father, but kept himself unaware of this idea. The source of the terrifying feelings instead became the bull under his bed, and he "displaced" this affect state (rage) from father to the bull.

Reaction formation, undoing, and isolation are frequently seen as a constellation, which often provides the ingredients of obsessive–compulsive neurotic mechanisms (Kessler, 1966). The formation of these mechanisms was clearly developed in Fred. Similarly, the mechanisms of projection and displacement are often seen in conjunction, and they form the basis for phobias, which were also a part of Fred's pathology.

III. Superego Assessment

From the preceding clinical material, Fred could be seen as a youngster "weighted down" by his superego. There was a very clear struggle with his aggressive drives, for which Fred used a variety of defenses. These impulses activated his superego responses. He appeared to have a harsh and hypercritical superego as well as a demanding one (he lived up to very high standards of nonaggressive behavior).

There were a number of powerful sources that fueled his superego development. His strong aggressive and anal drives had contributed to building the severe nature of his superego. Fred also appeared to have identified with his strict, obsessional father. He additionally needed to deny these drives, because his father had reacted so strongly when he had expressed them.

Fred's troubling superego appeared in a number of ways. He was beset by his "worries" and bad thoughts. He expressed a good deal of guilt (for example, the spot of blood on the driveway), and he feared punishment (the animals of the Sagebrook woods would attack him).

IV. Genetic–Dynamic Formulation

The central problem that Fred exhibited was conflict with his aggressive drives. He appeared to have reached the phallic level of development (competition theme) but primarily regressed to an anal structure. At the point of evaluation the therapist saw the defenses and character traits associated with anal conflicts—reaction formation (he was compliant, good, etc.) and orderliness (he was attempting to control his internal aggression).

There were a number of significant factors that had contributed to Fred's preoedipal struggles with his aggression. The major factor had been the father's sadism and uncontrollable rage expressed against Fred. The father's defensive style (his obsession, preoccupation with dirt) had also contributed to Fred's choice of defenses through identification with his father. His mother had also influenced his development. She appeared to have had difficulty handling Fred's early aggression and had allowed too much expression of his early rage. There was also a question of whether the mother had been depressed during Fred's early years. Perhaps she had been unable to provide for him in other ways as well.

In Fred's history, he appeared to express his early rage directly and impulsively with his siblings and in nursery school. His behavior problems were also accompanied by anxieties, especially separation anxiety (early fears of abandonment as a punishment). In early latency, he became well behaved but severely symptomatic. When his superego was fully formed and his ego became strengthened by maturation, he became able to contain his impulses. However, he spent an inordinate amount of psychic energy defending against awareness of his internal aggressive life. This was a youngster dominated by his neurosis at the time of his evaluation.

Diagnostically, Fred illustrated problems of a youngster who had developed an obsessional neurosis. How can we distinguish between patients with obsessional neurosis and those with pathologies such as borderline disorder or psychosis? The distinguishing feature is the quality of the child's ego functioning. Neurotic youngsters, like Fred, are well endowed, and their egos function on a high level. This example can be compared with the case of Matthew (Chapter 8), who used obsessional mechanisms within a borderline disorder. The primitive nature of his thinking and defense structure will be evident.

V. Treatment Recommendations

Residential treatment was recommended because of the ongoing severe problems at home, particularly the pathology of the father. Earlier outpatient attempts had not proved fruitful. In addition, uncovering psychotherapy was recommended to help Fred deal with his "intolerable" underlying aggressive impulses.

COURSE OF TREATMENT
Clinical Material: The Early Work

The impact of Fred's neurosis on his total personality became clearer in the first year of treatment. One could follow the debilitating effects of the primitive defense mechanisms Fred needed to employ: isolation, undoing, and magical thinking. The therapist could also witness the widespread suffering induced by his severely demanding superego.

After 4 months of treatment, the problem of aggression began to show itself directly, although not at first in the sessions. Fred took a sudden acute interest in war games in the cottage and became a subtle negative leader. Accidents began to crop up; there were a host of small injuries to younger peers. Attempts by staff to point out his behavior were met by protest. Fred insisted that everybody was just picking on him.

Fred began to report some very alien thoughts in the treatment hour. He had the impulse to throw the basketball at one of his cottage mates; he wanted to stab little Jeff with a knife. He was embarrassed in bringing forth these thoughts, but it might help to tell, he said, and he did have them. Simultaneously, a fear of rats appeared. He began seeing them around Sagebrook, particularly in the bushes. Some of them had strange shapes and seemed to be a hybrid of several small animals.

Some sadistic memories came into the hour. He described how he and a friend found the severed head of a deer in the woods. They hid it and returned daily to see all the white things crawling around. His already difficult reality behavior appeared aggravated by these recollections. His aggression toward his younger peers in the cottage mounted, and staff became concerned about their safety. Glen, an 8-year-old, was pushed off a swing; little Jeff, climbing at Whips Ledges Park, almost had a dangerous fall; David, recently returned from eye surgery, was hit by a ball that narrowly missed the operation site. Fred's aggression was at times out of control, and the cottage staff took many direct steps to isolate and supervise Fred.

At first Fred was totally unable to hear anything the therapist said about his behavior—for example, that these driven, angry feelings must come from something in his past. At the time of the David incident, Fred began complaining about his own eyes. He was sure the doctor had made an error in his recent glasses prescription, and he said, "A little mistake can cause a lot of damage to the eyes." The therapist pointed out that perhaps he was saying that his little mistake could have caused severe damage to David's eyes. Sudden strong guilt and anxiety came out in a rush; he was frightened that he was really going to hurt someone; he had even tried at other times to injure David, but he could not help it; it was so hard to stop. Confessing to many instances when he had had impulses to hurt others, he cried that he only wanted some control.

With direct cottage management, Fred brought more material to the hour. Little Jeff, he reported, fools everybody in the cottage, and he gets away with everything because all the staff think he is cute. If Jeff talks out, or even interrupts the prayer during supper (a major cottage offense), the counselors just giggle. He had seen Jeff steal cookies and put soap on toothbrushes. I could see, the therapist noted, that all of Fred's recent angry feelings must be connected to very strong jealous feelings. As jealousy was discussed, Fred's fear of rats spread dramatically, and he worried at night. Did he hear rats in the basement? Would they gnaw through the kitchen door and enter the cottage proper? When he began to doze off, he would awake with a start; he imagined they were nibbling on his cheek. Those notions caused an immediate outbreak of anxiety, and Fred wanted reality assurance: Did rats actually thrive at Sagebrook or not? The therapist began to interpret and connect these worries with thoughts of punishment that Fred was erecting against himself. He noted that the conscience part of Fred devised fears because he felt he was so terrible.

Fred's jealousy had its roots at home. Fred felt that he had lost his place in the family. He described how his room had been given to his sister and his furniture was now in the attic. He had a runaway dream: He reached home, and when he looked through a window, he saw Brad, his youngest brother, and his mother alone on the couch. He expressed an unusual amount of sadness, the first major affect of his treatment. He felt so outside, so left out and alone, and the therapist wondered whether little Jeff and Glen in the cottage had not come to represent the brother from home. The ability, at this point, to link the cottage situation affectively with his feelings about home and family and to understand some of the meaning of his aggression was a source of relief. There was a marked abatement of his fear of animals and general anxiety, as well as a marked decrease in his rage toward his peers.

Touching on Fred's aggressiveness gave both Fred and the therapist some awareness of the amount of sadism within him. Fred himself was quickly becoming aware of how profoundly his "inside feelings" and "inside thoughts" (as he and his therapist came to call them) were affecting his life. His rational ego witnessed to what lengths he could be driven and to what degrees he could conceive thoughts that punished himself. He was becoming more interested in what the therapist could do ultimately to restore order and provide relief, and there seemed to be a growing strength in the working alliance.

At times during the first year it was striking to see the quick escalation of anxiety and the sudden elaboration of symptoms. Fred's use of and belief in magic and omnipotence were impressive, especially at holiday time.

"Holiday time" was a cultural phenomenon at Sagebrook, beginning in November and lasting through Christmas. During this highly charged period the anticipation and anxieties about contact with family often become focalized and acted out.

We noticed early in November that Fred was making special long-distance calls to his home, pleading with his parents to make some extra weekend visits. If money or expenses were a problem, he suggested they use *his* bank account at home. He had to see them. During sessions, when the therapist noted his recent desperation, he expressed great anxiety. He had been increasingly concerned that his parents did not want to visit him at all. He was suspicious about the last postponed visit. Yes, he had received a postcard from his father in Oklahoma (where his father had to conduct some business that month), but he felt that despite the evidence of the postmark, the card had somehow really been mailed from home in Iowa. His parents just did not want to come. On other monthly visits he had kept track of the time they spent with him, and it seemed to be growing shorter. There had been many signs, he felt, that they did not want to stay. The therapist slowly began to wonder whether the reverse might not be true: Perhaps there was a part within Fred that did not want to see his parents.

How does a therapist make a judgment that the manifest content a patient presents (e.g., Fred's concern that his parents were rejecting) serves an important defensive function? The therapist was not aware of any real change in parental attitude. Fred's concern seemed increasingly irrational (e.g., he had received a card from his father from Oklahoma, but he felt it really had come from home in Iowa). The therapist was then led to try to work out what could be internally producing this concern in Fred. A plausible hypothesis was that Fred was defending against his own aggressive, rejecting impulses toward his parents and using the mechanism of projection by attributing his impulses to them.

After some initial denial, Fred became much more conscious of his aggressive feelings. For several days he became preoccupied with knives, long kitchen knives that he had seen both at home and at Sagebrook. He could not help some of the thoughts he had, he protested. He thought of stabbing the therapist, of plunging the knife into him; he just could not stop his killing thoughts. Because Fred was so frightened by such thoughts, the therapist conveyed acceptance of these ideas and encouraged him to elaborate. (The direct retaliatory fears came quickly. He became afraid to leave the therapist's office, fearing that he would be stabbed in the hallway.) About a week before the November parent visit, Fred began making unusual mistakes at school. He was beside himself with anxiety over his error. He had had a perfect spelling paper, with one exception. He had substituted the work "bury" for the word "berry." His associations were to a tool set his parents had given him. One day he buried it in the Sagebrook woods, and when he had returned to get it, it had been taken. Maybe he had wanted to get rid of it. The following day he left the "d" out of the word "hundred," and with much anxiety he had the thought that "d" stood for "dead"—"bury the dead." He then confessed some of his preoccupations: he feared his parents would never make it to Sagebrook and would have an accident on the road. He himself commented (intellectually) that this could be an aggressive thought on his part, but it was also (feelingly) a dreaded fear. Fred worried each day that he would make other spelling mistakes as the week wore on, and the therapist interpreted that he feared thought mistakes. Perhaps a lethal killing thought would mistakenly slip out.

In this period of time, a new level of participation emerged in Fred. The reason for this was that Fred was again experiencing intense anxiety and dread, and that he already had experienced relief when he had conveyed his thoughts in his therapy. Although this was a productive period, it is important to understand that the pace of therapy generally ebbs and flows. There were often significant periods of time (weeks) where little was learned or understood.

When the therapist prepared Fred for the fact that he would be gone Thanksgiving Day, Fred had an interesting reaction. Even though he had known the therapist would take the day off, he could not really believe this would happen. Further, if the therapist really missed a session, Fred knew he could not avoid having killing thoughts about him. Fantasies spilled out: The therapist was caught in a snowbank or consumed by lung cancer. During this period, when Fred fearfully asked whether the therapist thought he could be a real "murderer," they began to work on the magic, omnipotent quality of thoughts. He had many killing thoughts and killing wishes, the therapist explained, and he acted as though these thoughts could really hurt. Just as when he was little, he now mixed up his thoughts and deeds. If he angrily thought the therapist would die of cancer, he feared that the idea would happen. This was an old idea that had been strong when he was little and that he still kept. But everyone has a whole variety of thoughts and feelings all the time. (Many rat fears and eating inhibitions were plaguing Fred during this period. He was down to drinking milk as his only food at one point.)

Several weeks before his parents visited in December, Fred began counting. At a children's concert at the music hall he counted the leaves in the decoration on the ceiling, somehow, to keep the roof from falling in. He counted the colored glass panes in the chapel at Sagebrook, again to keep the roof intact. And each day he counted and recounted the number of days left before his parents would come. Yes, it was magic! If he stopped, and he could not, his parents might die on the trip. He then quietly discussed all the plans he had ruminated about, should that event occur. He would live with his grandparents in Florida, or with his aunt in Chicago, or with another aunt in South Bend. As visiting day approached, he had many "nervous" feelings and his neck became stiff. The stiff neck, we finally understood, was the result of a struggle. He fought his desire to look out the window at the passing cars. Would he have a lethal look? He kept his parents safe by stiffly looking forward at the therapist. With this awareness, Fred fought his fears and allowed himself to look out the window. His parents arrived safe and sound.

As we anticipated the Christmas holidays, new material appeared in the transference. Fred's killing thoughts toward the therapist were active and prominent. The therapist made him feel helpless every day when he was kept waiting before his hour started. Slowly, memories about home came, and they stirred up an enormous feeling of helplessness: the helpless feeling he had when he tried to get his mother's attention, but she only had time to play cards with Brad; the helpless feeling when his father started yelling or when his father threw his sister's shoes or silverware across the living room; the total helplessness when his father stood over him with a face red with anger. The therapist spoke with Fred about the only means a little helpless boy *could have* in coping with such situations and attempted some reconstruction: A little boy overpowered could get back only by magic. He would make many killing, hurting, getting-even ideas, and these were the "inside" getting-back thoughts that came out now. He had never had help, and this old kind of anger never grew up.

Not only during holiday time but throughout the period of treatment, there was a significant problem with Fred's loyalty feelings. The many contrasts that Fred saw between Sagebrook and home provoked constant guilt, for Sagebrook often did so much better. The more he liked his therapist, the more he responded to the staff's interest and concern, and the more he witnessed their efforts to erect effective controls, the greater became his outrage and disappointment in his years at home.

This clinical material highlights several aspects of Fred's treatment that will be discussed: the nature of his early *resistance* and the *interventions* by the therapist dealing with his presenting conflicts.

How was Fred's resistance evident in this case? In his first year of treatment, Fred evidenced a number of ego resistances in his sessions. Early in treatment, as Fred had begun to show some of his aggressive problems with peers in the cottages, he brought "alien thoughts" about his cottage mates into the sessions. These had included the thought of "throwing a basketball" at a peer and "stabbing little Jeff." These observations had been made in great detail, and as though observed from a distance. The therapist became aware of the defenses (ego resistances) of *intellectualization* and *isolation of affect* that Fred used prominently. He pointed out that when Fred brought the ideas of hurting others, he discussed them in a very detailed but detached and intellectual way. The therapist suggested that perhaps Fred was afraid of allowing himself to feel angry, and he therefore needed to push these feelings away by his special way of describing things. Because the therapist understood the purpose of this ego resistance, he interpreted its function to Fred. The major initial goal was to slowly help Fred come closer to his internal aggressive life, which he actively pushed away. The defense interpretations would help to erode the repressive barrier that Fred created against his affects.

Somewhat later in this period of work, the therapist focused on other ego resistances. At holiday time, Fred was worried that his parents would not want to visit. The therapist understood the mechanism of "projection," putting one's forbidden impulses outside and attributing them to another person. When the therapist made the defense interpretation, "Perhaps the reverse was true, and there was a part in Fred that did not want to see his parents," the therapist helped Fred to focus on his own aggressive impulses. This allowed Fred to experience subsequent aggressive thoughts of kitchen knives and death preoccupations in regard to his parents.

During this intense holiday time, Fred was driven to count the leaves in the ceiling decoration at the music hall in order to keep the ceiling from falling in. The therapist was aware of the mechanism of "undoing," which Fred used prominently. Fred was compelled to act (count the leaves correctly) to magically keep a disaster from happening (the roof from falling). The therapist described this driven, repeated act. The therapist spoke to several aspects of Fred's driven behavior. He seemed very concerned about making a mistake and tried to correct it by counting. But what could the mistake be? Fred worried about the ceiling falling in, but did he have to "undo" some other disaster that he feared? Perhaps it was the fear that his thoughts could hurt his parents. Again, in the early work with Fred, the therapist helped him to understand how his ego worked, how he used a variety of defenses to ward off affects.

In the preceding clinical material with Fred, we can follow the sequence of the intervention process. An example of this occurs early in Fred's treatment, as his good behavior changes in the cottage and he "accidently" roughs up some of his peers. The initial *confrontation* is brought by the cottage staff. They make explicit to Fred's ego that he is acting aggressively with his peers and trying to hurt them. This is brought clearly to his attention, although Fred does not overtly acknowledge his "accidents" to his peers. Fred does bring the aggressive feelings into his treatment hour and describes a number of his destructive impulses (toward David, Glen, etc.). As Fred described these incidents, the therapist was able to clarify (to bring the phenomenon into sharper focus). This aggressive behavior was not aimed at peers in general but specifically at the younger children. The aggressive impulses thus had greater specificity. When the focus became the little children, and particularly the youngster Jeff whom Fred described as loved by the cottage for his cuteness, there was an opportunity to make an *interpretation*.

The function of an *interpretation* is to give meaning to behavior, which is controlled by unconscious processes. The therapist noted that "Fred was so angry because he felt very jealous." Although this interpretation was rather simple, Fred had had no idea why he felt the rage. The motive for his anger was unconscious and repressed, and becoming aware of this dynamic brought back material about his family in the next few weeks.

Fred's rage/jealous feelings were painful to him, because they centered on his younger siblings at home, who he felt were loved by his parents, whereas he had been rejected. The motive for repression was to avoid this painful awareness. When the interpretation was made, these memories could become available to his consciousness. In the treatment he described that he currently felt displaced by his sister and brother, recalled his furniture being sent to the attic, dreamt that his mother and youngest brother Brad were close on the couch. As this material emerged, Fred experienced the affects of loss, rejection, rage, and killing wishes toward his young siblings.

The therapist then had an opportunity to *work through* the initial insight, to examine further meanings of the jealousy interpretation. For example, he noted with Fred that jealous feelings toward siblings experienced at a very young age quite often contain intense rage and killing ideas (e.g., "put the baby in the garbage"). These ideas can often be maintained when one grows up. In addition, there can be many new, similar situations that will trigger these early feelings. They now emerged in the "new family" with new "siblings" in the cottage at Sagebrook.

In considering this sequence, it is important to understand that the "jealousy" interpretation to Fred was a simple one. Beginning therapists often think that an interpretation must be profound to be effective and thus they bring many complex ideas to the child patient. In reality, simple ideas are usually most effective and more easily integrated by the child.

How do people change? Does the *insight* presented have any effect on Fred, and can we credit the therapist with a *"mutative interpretation"* (an interpretation that produces a change in symptoms)? This process did provide beginning relief for Fred (some fears and troubling dreams abated), and it can be understood in the following way. Although Fred repressed his rage and sadistic feelings, it was clear that he was experiencing unconscious guilt, and he lived with many fears of punishment from his surround. During the treatment process, he became more consciously and affectively aware of his "killing feelings" and great rage toward his peers. As he and the therapist attempted to understand his rage, insight provided a new perspective. These current sadistic feelings were manifestations of the old repressed feelings of his childhood when he had felt displaced by new siblings. These were typical "little boy" feelings, which he had to totally push away, and they had returned currently in unmodified form with the same intensity he had experienced as a younger child. The effect of this period of psychotherapy was to give these current and troubling feelings a new context for Fred. Rather than serving as evidence to himself that he was a murderous monster (his own harsh superego reaction), these feelings now had an understandable history and context that could ameliorate Fred's severe internal superego reaction. There was evidence of this change, as Fred could slowly allow more natural aggression in his daily behavior with peers (he was no longer always fair and good, with sudden "accidental" outbreaks), and his fears and terrors disappeared for a period of time. His aggressive feelings became increasingly more tolerable to him, and he did not need to have his conscience torture him for these feelings.

Clinical Material: The Later Work

Whereas the early part of Fred's treatment dealt primarily with his problems of aggression, it was not until well into the second year of treatment that sexual conflicts emerged clearly. Phallic urges and masturbation feelings appeared in a way that could be used in treatment.

At first Fred became preoccupied with the therapist's pipe smoking. He hoped the therapist would not be angry with him for his comment, he noted in preface, but he did feel it was a rather dirty habit. Did he know he could make himself sick? Hadn't the therapist read the medical reports about smoking? His father had stopped. The therapist mentioned that boys often thought about a therapist's habits when they were concerned about their own. When *his* habits were discussed, a "bad one" was discovered: Fred picked his nails. It gave him pleasure, but he would continue until his fingers became sore and painful. He could not stop even though his mother had told him to. He picked whenever he was bored, such as during his social study lecture each afternoon at school. With boredom came restlessness. Several days later, he solved the school dilemma. The restless, bored feeling completely vanished when he took notes and kept his hands busy. The therapist had to wonder what he thought idle hands might do.

The hand theme continued. He was having a daily debate now about washing his hands. Should he go and wash or not? He confessed to strange solutions. Sometimes he would eat a meal with several days' dirt on his hands (he would make believe he washed), and other times he found himself rewashing already clean hands just to make himself feel better. This habit had started about a year before he came to Sagebrook. He had stuck himself with a pencil, and it had left a lead mark on his palm. He had become concerned about blood poisoning and had tried to wash the spot out. Since then, there had been many times when the hand-washing idea became strong. Recently, at night, as he lay in bed he got the bored, restless feeling, and then got up and washed his hands, experiencing relief. He was interested in the therapist's comments. The therapist suggested that some "inside" struggle must be going on at night. Did he need to wash away something dirty?

He was plagued with many disgusting thoughts. He was troubled by smashing animals and had a recurring memory of a squirrel hit by a bus. He could not forget a science film at school. The heart of a dog was removed during an operation. Fred found it hard to look at the dissected rabbit in his biology class, and he also worried about how frequently he had been getting colds during the winter. The therapist noted with him his preoccupation with injury and his concerns about his body, tentatively suggesting that boys worried sometimes about their "habits." The worry that habits could hurt them physically was a very common concern. For several days Fred told of a recurring dream: He was climbing high on a roof (sometimes at home, sometimes in the cottage at Sagebrook), and suddenly a shingle broke and he fell. Through his association it emerged that the high climbing was really being alive and manly (he always wanted to climb, even mountains), but something in him made it all feel very dangerous. (Look at what happened when you tried!)

A very strong avoidance set in, the first major avoidance. Fred became quiet and sullen. His treatment hour was the gloomiest hour of the day, and he could not wait until it was over. Each hour he waited for the time to go by, and for the first time, he came late to his sessions. The therapist began to interpret the reversal and suggested that Fred was really expecting him to stop treatment. He feared the therapist would just get disgusted with his disgusting thoughts and disgusting habits and throw him out. These seemed to be his "outcast feelings."

With great shame, he finally told the therapist of his wetting symptoms. He had long since stopped wetting his bed, but under certain circumstances during the day several drops came out, and he could not control this. Most people, he thought, controlled themselves at age 3 or 4. No one else had a problem like it. Slowly he described the following situations that produced the wetting: just before being tested in the gym (racing or rope climbing), writing on the blackboard in front of the class, acting in a community night play at Sagebrook. He was really frightened of his forthcoming Confirmation. What would happen if he completely wet his pants during the service? He could begin to feel that performing in some way made him very anxious. The therapist noted that just when he was to show some ability or his intelligence or physical strength, another part of him suddenly became broken or defective.

The therapist then drew a number of things together: Fred's worry about bad habits he could not stop, his need to clean his hands, his fear of bodily injury, and his sense of danger when he felt manly. It was noted that with boys his age, these feelings were often brought up when they had a struggle with their sexual feelings and fought their strong urges to touch and play with their penis.

He then told the therapist that recently he had been masturbating a great deal. Fred related that he had always been worried that something was wrong with his penis, because he had wet for years. His penis and groin area hurt him a lot recently, and sometimes he had stabbing pains. He had heard that boys had growing pains, and he wondered openly if his bad "habits" could hurt the body in some way. Fred and the therapist came to understand more clearly that his compulsive need to touch himself was to find out repeatedly whether he was still all right.

A torrent of sexual questions came out, questions about body structure, about his new external and internal physical changes. He thought about the differences between men and women, about pregnancy, and he had concerns about his semen, ejaculation, and his short stature. There seemed to be much relief in this expression. For a while there was relief from the compulsive need to masturbate and the disturbing wetting symptom. The therapist felt that Fred had taken an important step; he could look directly at phallic material.

In his last year of treatment, another aspect of phallic threat was explored. When masculine urges were associated with achievement in schoolwork, Fred reacted with an inhibition of activity and competition.

During Fred's final year at Sagebrook, he began to look much more like an adolescent. He was changing physically, developed an interest in girls, and participated actively in all sports. He also began, however, to have some major trouble in junior high school, but the source was not the earlier ritualistic checking and rechecking of his work. He just "neglected" work that he could do; he did not fail but did less than he was capable of. This inhibition was rooted in his competitive feelings toward his father. Slowly Fred and the therapist could come to understand more about the effect of his early sadomasochistic interplay with his father.

Fred now openly deprecated his father. His father was successful in business, he felt, without even working for it. He took 3 hours for lunch, gabbed all the time with people, and his grandfather had really set him up in the business anyway. He knew his father's pretentions; he brought his portfolio home but never worked from it. His father called himself "president," but it was really a one-man company. Besides, Fred himself would be different. He was going to have a profession and help people. When news came from home that his father had been elected chairman of the United Fund or appointed to the executive council of the local Republican Party, Fred always felt they could have found someone more suitable.

Fred's relationship with his therapist changed markedly, as did his overall adjustment at Sagebrook. He began to wonder about the therapist's competence. He felt he was being helped much more by the cottage staff, just by talking with them for 10 minutes each day. Words like "stupid" and "ignoramus" began to come into his vocabulary, and he became much more direct and brave. Slowly the hours became an enormous and immensely pleasurable flight. Yes, he certainly had thoughts, but he definitely was not going to share them with the therapist. He became sarcastic. If, for instance, using his material, the therapist discussed some anxiety about his health, Fred might say he had a great new solution. He was going to take Carter's one-a-day vitamin pills. He came late for an appointment and entered with a pleased smile. He got up and left abruptly just when the therapist would begin some "profound" interpretation. He would outargue and outfox every move and now reported that he was going to be a famous trial lawyer. And this was so pleasurable and wonderful he felt he would never stop.

In the cottage he talked with peers about how much of a "clod" Chethik (the therapist) was, and he had the boys laughing at the clumsiness of the therapeutic staff, questioning the logic of every rule and regulation imposed. Slowly, the therapist began working with Fred to show him how he was fighting his father in the guise of other people. He seemed to be reliving a past relationship with his father, with one difference. Before, when he was little, he could not fight back or stand up to his father's anger. Now he seemed to be fighting and expressing a long-withheld rebellion that had been within him for many years.

Fred, in his retaliation, found many victims. He began to take advantage of the weaker boys in the cottage; he rented his baseball glove for 25 cents per hour to a very passive boy; he made bets with another helpless child, bets that he had to win. All of this was justified, he claimed, because he had always been made a victim. He described how the cottage staff resorted to physical punishment when they were frustrated. He resolved that "if I get it, I am going to give it back." He recalled how humiliated he had been on a recent home visit when his uncle had switched off his program to watch a football game. He had had no resources; he had been helpless. Here the therapist noted with Fred that these feelings were emerging so strongly because he had once felt so helpless and little with his father. Now, however, instead of being in the frightened role, he had become the tormenter. Even though he felt terribly guilty about his behavior, somehow it was safer for him not to be the victim. This was his way of warding off his memories, and it kept him from reexperiencing the old humiliations he had felt.

He was just overcoming some of his past humiliations, Fred said. He had always been short, and as a youngster he used to play baseball with a group of older boys. They had called him "stupid" and "shrimp," and while he was batting they used to make him swing at balls over his head. Now he was becoming a good ballplayer, and he was determined to become a professional. One day, those same boys who had attacked him would be shocked when he became a star. Yet he was still very concerned that he would never grow adequately. If at age 18 he was too small to reach the gas pedals of a car and so unable to drive, he would be so angry that his anger would never end!

He came in hopelessly and terribly beaten one day because his wetting had started again. The therapist wondered with Fred how much, no matter what he did in reality, he still felt like the "little drip." Inside, from his memories, he always compared himself with his father. His father was the big gun, but he remained the little leaky one. Until he could know more of the past, a part inside of him would find a way to humiliate him.

Slowly memories of his beatings emerged, and with much affect. His father had chased him, and he had run because he was terrified. His father had used a doubled-up belt, and he would hit him sometimes without stopping. Often before the beating started, his father just stared at him, his face red all over and his eyes seeming to bulge. He used to have a compelling wish during a beating that he would be dead and come to life only after the beating because he so dreaded the pain. He used to become numb and paralyzed; he wanted to say something, but his vocal chords would not work. He remembered the scene of the dog in *Call of the Wild*, the one that was beaten with a club until his master was exhausted. How the dog tried to think of something else! Many times he felt his parents were like the Romans, throwing him to the lions and getting great pleasure from it and cheering wildly. Again and again, Fred came back to his reaction: the numbness, paralysis, dreamlike feelings he experienced. He said on several occasions that when he remembered what had happened to him when he was little, he could now see why he was so angry with the world. When he was young, he never stopped getting into trouble, always provoking his mother and brothers and thus invoking further beatings.

Fred's descriptions of his beating experiences helped us to understand a number of patterns in Fred's behavior. One aspect was how he constantly seemed to invite force. Often in his present reality, Fred described parallels. He tended at times to neglect his homework until the cottage staff was looking over his shoulder. On several occasions he let his schoolwork lie undone until the teacher insisted that he do his work in after-school special help classes. At times, as we worked on this material, Fred stayed away from his sessions. He seemed intent on getting the therapist to act, to have him escorted from the cottage, or to threaten the treatment in some way. The therapist could now begin to work with Fred to show him how his wish for the beatings was as strong as ever, and that in many ways he continued to lead the life of a young child with a dominating father. He tried to provoke the therapist to take action in the treatment situation, as he did in other facets of his life. He repeatedly became humiliated, but part of him wanted to get to the point where people overpowered him again. He seemed to have very mixed feelings about the beatings, as if part of him had come to enjoy them.

Another important element of the beatings was how frightening it became for Fred to be active. We saw evidence of this in Fred's problems with his schoolwork. Sometimes he was unable to do his homework, especially when he had a large load. He was afraid to study too hard, as it brought on headaches. His fantasies were that the stress of the work would affect his brain, would ruin his brain and make it deteriorate. He was often ambivalent about his exams; there was a desire to fail them and do poorly so that in life he could be a failure. If worse came to worse, he could always work for his father. In school he would take copious notes, usually more than the other students, but often he would completely neglect reviewing them before an exam. He could not hand in an insect collection for his science project. The most repugnant part of the assignment was that he would have to mount the insects, and he did not feel he could "stick the pins in." In summary, Fred was very frightened of his ambition and drive, and part of him needed to keep himself impotent. The therapist worked with Fred to show him how a similar "paralysis" (similar to the paralysis associated with his beatings) seemed to develop when he needed to perform. Now he seemed to become paralyzed in his learning situation. He became terrified whenever he needed to show what he could do. Where could this come from? Slowly Fred and the therapist came to understand that he had interpreted much of his father's wrath as an attack on his activity. They knew, for example, that he had been beaten for his house climbing, and this was his young masculine pursuit. He had also been beaten for his wetting, and he had come to feel that this was for his genital and exciting manly thoughts. Now, in every current manly and achieving area, he became "paralyzed" because he thought he would be attacked. And, of course, his ambition was strongly linked with the killing revenge on his father. Neglect kept his father safe. This was the major area of work before termination.

In the preceding clinical material, Fred began to experience a significant *transference* reaction. The earlier conforming youngster was now angry and belittling of his therapist. Chethik was a "clod" and "ignoramus" and the object of scorn and humiliation. One could certainly say that the quality of the relationship with the therapist had changed, and Fred was experiencing affects toward the therapist that did not befit the relationship.

When the therapist understood that this change in the relationship was a manifestation of transference, he felt he could slowly bring this to Fred's awareness (as described earlier) because this would be beneficial to him. Despite his new anger with the therapist, Fred had a good therapeutic alliance with him and a history of meaningful work together when changes had occurred. The attachment that was developed within the alliance would help Fred gain some distance as patient, and therapist explored the current anger in the transference.

What was being transferred? What was being repeated in regard to significant persons of the past, displaced into the present? Fred had had a significant sadomasochistic relationship with his father that was a very significant factor in his pathology, it had reemerged in the present in action but not in awareness. Fred sought to justify his demeaning of the therapist—he felt the therapist had wasted Fred's time, and he was therefore a major ignoramus. One can see some of the dangers to the therapy as the transference emerges, particularly the danger of gratification. As a little boy, Fred felt helpless and suffered much humiliation at the hands of the powerful father-bull. In demeaning the present authority, there was intense gratification in living out a revenge opportunity to undo the past. Now, at last, he could put down and humiliate a major authority. Insight brought by the therapist would destroy the immediate opportunity—therefore, Fred noted with pleasure that he could out-argue and out-fox the therapist, and he would never stop. Other dangers were Fred's fears and discomfort as his rage emerged. He naturally feared that the therapist would retaliate and react to his provocations, and the danger would feel immense because the fears stemmed from the childhood situation with his father. For a significant period, Fred did not listen to or take in any of the therapist's comments.

When a therapist is under attack, there are natural internal counterreactions that he or she often needs to handle. Is the patient justified in his assessment? Am I really a "clod" and an "ignoramus"? There can often be a blow to one's therapeutic narcissism and self-esteem. There is often significant counter-rage and frustration. How can this patient do this when I have invested so much? These are some of the natural internal thoughts and struggles until the therapist can understand why the material arises. These counterreactions are typically more intense in the new and inexperienced therapist whose professional self-assurance is naturally fragile, but they remain the internal response of experienced therapists as well.

Over a period of time, the therapist's *interventions* became effective, and we can follow the process of the uncovering interventions. Initially the therapist *confronted* the patient—he noted that the relationship had changed, inasmuch as Fred was fighting and angry all the time in the hour, and questioned whether this behavior was justified or coming from somewhere else. As Fred continued to berate the therapist, further *clarification* was made explicit to Fred's ego. The therapist brought into greater focus the interplay between himself and Fred. Fred seemed to need to humiliate the therapist, as though he was taking revenge for some major experience of the past. Fred commented that this might be true, but that the situation would continue forever. The timing of an interpretation is important. The quality of the transference should be established and lived out to some extent (because gratification needs to be experienced, and its inappropriateness more fully established).

The therapist then slowly made the transference *interpretation*, giving unconscious meaning to this fighting behavior with the therapist. Fred seemed to be engaged in a fighting relationship with the therapist (and other "authorities"), and it had the same form of his old relationship with his father in which he had felt humiliated and helpless. These past memories always made him feel uncomfortable, and he smoldered inside. Now they were reemerging, but with one important change. Earlier he was a child and could not fight back, but currently he had reversed the process, and he now was the aggressor and humiliator. At first, there was little overt acknowledgment, but Fred did describe tormenting his peers. He subsequently discussed the humiliation by his uncle, and there was a temporary return of a humiliating daytime wetting symptom he had had as a child, which brought back more of the past. Slowly he gained access to many memories of the beatings by his father, as he had described earlier, with the affects of terror, paralysis, and helpless rage.

In the process of *working through* (the elaborated process of examining the implications of an insight), Fred and his therapist sorted out how this early intense conflict with his father had shaped significant aspects of his personality and how he was currently affected by this history. Three themes were discovered. (1) They focused on how this past trauma had established a reservoir of rage/hatred within Fred that could easily be provoked by current authorities. (2) They also identified the patterns of current provocation. The clinical material illustrated the pervasiveness of Fred's current need to invite force. In treatment, he missed sessions and provoked the cottage staff to bring him to his appointments; in the cottage, his aggressive actions brought sanctions; in school, the teachers reacted to him for his lack of preparation. In an unconscious way, Fred "set up" authorities to "come down" on him, and he thereby relived the provocation–humiliation pattern with the "fathers" of today. (3) Similarly, Fred was terrified of his active–assertive behavior. He feared using his mind and intellectual skills, because this meant competition, even though he was currently encouraged to achieve. The past wrath of his father for assertive behavior continued to instill fear and inhibition. These themes and further insights (the process of working through) developed from the original uncovering of the early struggle between father and son. The working-through process took a 6-month period.

Fred was discharged from Sagebrook, and he continued to live away from home. He attended a coeducational boarding school with high academic standards. In follow-up contacts, the therapist learned that he was performing well academically, was free of any obsessional symptoms, and seemed to be making a rather typical heterosexual adjustment. He was quite assertive with teachers and peers and internally felt relatively untroubled.

The concepts of the psychotherapy process discussed in this chapter are further explained with respect to a variety of cases in subsequent chapters.

SUMMARY

This chapter has introduced the neurotic child. The aspect of an emotional disturbance that makes it a neurosis is that it is based on internalized conflict, conflict between different parts of the personality within. A major struggle evident with Fred was the conflict between his aggressive impulses (id) and his conscience (superego). This internal conflict led to repression/defenses and an outbreak of symptoms in latency.

The neurosis is generally believed to be a benign emotional disturbance (Kessler, 1966) because it responds most favorably to psychotherapy. In this case presentation, a variety of insight-oriented techniques have been described. For the neurotic child, the past is unconscious (repressed), yet it lives on as though it were real in situations akin to those of the past. The "uncovering" process of psychotherapy allows the child patient to see how his past distorts his current reality. Because neurotic patients are generally intact in areas that are conflict-free, the insights they gain about "distorting" the current situation help them alter their behavior. When Fred gained the "insight" that his rage toward his younger cottage mates reflected his feelings about his family as a child, the intensity of his current aggression abated.

BIBLIOGRAPHY

Erikson, F. (1963). *Childhood and Society*. New York: W. W. Norton.

Greenson, R. (1967). *The Technique and Practice of Psychoanalysis*. New York: International Universities Press.

Kessler, J. (1966). *Psychopathology of Childhood*. Englewood Cliffs, NJ: Prentice Hall.

Langs, R. (1973). *The Technique of Psychoanalytic Psychotherapy*, Vol. 1. New York: Jason Aronson.

Nagera, H. (1976). *Obsessional Neurosis*. New York: Jason Aronson.

Sandler, J., Holder, A., & Dare, C. (1973). *The Patient and the Analyst*. New York: International Universities Press.

Sander, J., Kennedy, H., & Tyson, R. (1980). *The Technique of Child Psychoanalysis: Discussion with Anna Freud*. Cambridge, MA: Harvard University Press.

7

∼

Treatment of
Character Pathology

Before one begins to think about the process of treatment of character pathology, it is helpful to understand some of the theory of character and character pathology. How would one define the concept of character itself? Fenichel (1945) has described it as the consistent, organized part of the personality, the habitual mode of adjustment that the ego has developed. Others have similar concepts. For example, character is defined as the basic core of the personality (Abend, 1983), or those aspects that denote the individuality of its possessor (Stein, 1969). In summation, character is the personal stamp of an individual, which has a regularity, a stability, and an enduring quality.

Character traits and neurotic symptoms have often been contrasted. Character traits are typically described as "ego-syntonic" (qualities felt by the individual to be an intrinsic part of the self), whereas neurotic symptoms are described as "ego-alien" (qualities felt by the individual as something to get rid of and in the way). For an individual, his character traits are so basic to him that they are taken for granted. Neurotic symptoms are usually a cause for complaint and seen as a foreign body. For example, Fred (Chapter 6) had a number of obsessional neurotic symptoms. He had to "check and

A version of this chapter, "The Defiant Ones," by M. Chethik, was published in *Journal of Clinical Social Work*, Spring 1987, Vol. 15, No. 1, pp. 35–42.

recheck" his math; he had to be so conscious about not losing his place as he read that he could not concentrate on the content. But he was pained by these symptoms and wanted to be rid of them. He therefore felt they were on the periphery of his personality and not part of the "real Fred," who should be without these bothersome qualities. In contrast, the fighting and general belligerence of Mark (Chapter 1) was much closer to a character trait (a general counter-phobic stance). Mark was proud of his "lion feelings," his toughness and "masculinity." This quality in his personality protected him against any imagined onslaught from the outside. His hypermasculinity was felt by Mark to be his essence and central to him. Again, character traits are described as ego-syntonic in contrast with neurotic symptoms, which are experienced as ego-dystonic or ego-alien.

When we turn to children and the concept of character, we must take into account the ongoing development process. Character is a result of a relatively completed developmental and integrative process, which is not fully consolidated until all major ego and superego functions are stabilized (Abend, 1983). This is achieved, some authors note, by the end of adolescence. Nonetheless, it is clear that children are in the process of developing character traits, and we usually describe these qualities as "on the way" to character formation or character pathology, rather than fully completed.

The term "character pathology" or "character disorder" is used when a habitual mode of adjustment an individual has developed has taken a pathological turn. Typically, when most people think of character disorders, the image conjured up is that of the antisocial personality. Actually, there are *two* major categories of character pathology: the impulse-ridden character disorder and the neurotic character (Fenichel, 1945).

The "impulse-ridden character pathology group" is defined as those individuals whose habitual mode of adjustment is instinct expressive, and indeed, it does describe the typical antisocial personality. In these children or adults, their egos habitually allow the expression of immediate pleasures. They cannot delay gratification, and their consciences have not effectively built the reactions and inhibitions that one would expect in the course of development. These individuals become the psychopathic adults, the addictive personalities (alcoholics, drug users, etc.), and individuals who have major social conflicts (impulsive aggression, fighting, destructiveness, stealing, etc.). In a metapsychological appraisal, these people evidence a fragile ego, have limited defense formation, require restraints to be imposed from the outside, do not accept the limits of reality, and typically evince little sublimation potential (the ability to work productively) (Michaels & Stiver, 1965).

In contrast, the neurotic character group is delineated by the fact that their habitual mode of adjustment was dominated by massive conflict in their development. Typically, these adults and children develop a *fixed and pervasive defensive structure*, which permeates the entire personality. Thus, a youngster who is "on the way" to becoming an obsessional character (one type of neurotic character) would have these obsessional qualities "spread" into every aspect of his functioning. In the obsessional character, the control mechanisms would not only be evident in his rituals or obsessions but would also be found in his posture, bearing, and physical gait. His speech may be rigid and precise. Thus, the obsessional qualities would not be localized in various symptoms but would be extensively expressed throughout the personality.

In general, the treatment of individuals with character pathology is more difficult than treatment of neurotic patients. A therapist's confronting the behavior or qualities that are part of the character is typically very threatening to these patients, because these qualities are central to their functioning. They often feel that their whole sense of "being" or sense of self is at stake. Therapeutic alliances are thus difficult to build, and there is particularly strong resistance to the recognition of their basic pathology.

This chapter focuses on the most typical kind of character problem found in childhood, in which there is a mixture of impulse-ridden and neurotic character elements. The most common referrals to psychiatric and outpatient clinics for children are the fighting, defiant, and "out of control" youngsters who are very action oriented. This type of young patient exhibits trouble at home with discipline, problems with peers through provocation, and, characteristically, many behavior issues in school. Throughout his early years, this action discharge mode is often in evidence. A significant percentage of these children have potential character disorders—they are "on their way" to consolidating a permanent antisocial character pattern in adolescence or young adulthood.

In attempting to understand this group of children, Freud's (1937) discussion in *Analysis Terminable and Interminable* seems particularly relevant. He describes a group of adult patients for whom "quantitative factors" in their personality make treatment very difficult; they struggle with the *excessive strength* of their instincts because of constitutional factors or developmental experiences and find it much harder at every stage of development to "tame these instincts." He further discusses two major implications for development caused by this struggle. These patients characteristically have a *low threshold for frustration of instinctual wishes* and thereby tend toward immediate discharge of tension. Second, they have a low threshold for the tolerance of anxiety. Many of these aforementioned defiant children show problems with quantity of instinctual drive, low frustration, and problems in tolerating anxiety. These aspects in their development represent the impulse-ridden components of their character problems.

In addition, these youngsters also develop massive defensive structures. Particularly prominent is the mechanism of "identification with the aggressor" or the defense of "passive into active." The mechanisms are typically used in childhood, when the young, helpless child plays being the "boss" or "teacher" or powerful superhero. He copes with his feeling of helplessness (the natural state of many children) by temporarily turning passive into active, whereby he is the ruler or commander rather than the child who must comply.

From the developmental histories of these defiant youngsters, we can see that they use these particular mechanisms in a pervasive way. Often this emerges in the process of superego (conscience) development. In order to build the conscience, the child has to internalize the parental prohibitions. For such children, the parental inhibition stirs enormous anxiety, and they feel massively threatened, helpless, and weak. They "cope" with this threat by the mechanism of "identification with the aggressor"—they transfer themselves from the person being threatened to the person making the attack. They ward off being defenseless and helpless by becoming the attacker. This pattern becomes a vigorous and pervasive defensive mode that seems to permeate the whole personality.

The purpose of this chapter is to (1) describe these youngsters, (2) provide a diagnostic appraisal, (3) highlight some of the typical treatment problems, and (4) discuss techniques that have been developed to deal with the massive resistances these children employ. Fortunately, many such children have not fully developed the "armor plating of the personality" (Reich, 1963) that comes with time. Their defenses are not as solidified as those of the adult, and anxiety as an affect still remains therapeutically available. The principles of treatment with these children have a good deal of application to the treatment of character pathology in general.

These issues are discussed through the presentation of Roger L, a handsome, energetic, and extremely defiant late-latency-aged youngster.

ROGER: PRESENTING PICTURE, HISTORY, INITIAL SESSIONS

One was immediately impressed with Roger's precocious "macho" quality and his premature manliness. He had a swagger, a tough gait, and cursed easily and fluently in his initial meetings with his therapist, although he was only 10 years old. Roger was the middle child in a sibship of three; a sister was 2 years older, and a brother 4 years younger. He came from a middle-class, educated, professional family. His parents were concerned about their son's intense rages. For example, Roger reacted with fury to his father's demands: "Turn down the radio" would provoke a loud blasting of rock music; "Close the car window" would be met with an increase in the flow of air. Roger was often in trouble in school: He fought constantly, often losing out to older children, but always taking on a "dare." His fighting had led to detentions and a series of suspensions from school. He could provoke his teacher by greeting her with "Hi, stupid" as he entered the classroom in the morning. At age 10, the parents were already worried about his major attraction to the Lepke gang in the neighborhood, a group of young tough adolescents who were noted for their interest in drugs and minor vandalism. Generally the parents were strong, effective people, but with Roger, the father was often provoked into counter-rage (yelling, screaming), and the mother developed a placating, accommodating role to avoid trouble.

In the history, Roger was remembered as a very active baby, enjoyed by the family. As an energetic toddler, his mother found him hard to pursue at times, but although Roger was vigorous, he seemed happy and alert. He was, however, very frightened during the process of toilet training, especially avoiding the potty, and it took him 6 months to accomplish this task at 2½ years of age. His mother felt she was putting little pressure on Roger and was surprised by his struggle. Both parents thought it was striking that he became very frightened and somewhat alienated from his father at that time, and was particularly afraid of his father's deep, loud, booming voice and his mustache. However, by age 3½, the previously described pattern of defiance began and generally spread. Roger now did not fear his father; he defied him. He fought the daily demands with a characteristic "No, I won't. You can't make me." Accompanying Roger's counterphobic stance during the years were shortened periods of symptom formation. Sleep problems, enuresis, and tics were evident periodically, lasting, at times, for several months.

From the onset, Roger knew he was coming to see a therapist because of his "bad temper." He described how he was beset, however, by hosts of classmates who provoked him, and one could only expect that he would defend himself. Similarly, his brother and sister provoked him, and he was forced to retaliate. It was clear that as he described his active forms of revenge, a characteristic smile of pleasure came over his face.

He was angry at his mother, who was always hovering and worrying about him and who thought he was terrible. He wished she would "just get off his back." With pleasure he described some of the boys of the Lepke gang; he felt much pride that he was a fully accepted member although he was the youngest. He spoke of the huge collection of *Playboy* magazines the group had accumulated.

Roger told his therapist, during the evaluation sessions, that he was not going to see him. He was boring and probably charged too much, and he could not make him stay. He ended these initial sessions, however, by relating a recent nightmare—a dream in which his mother's severed head was rolling in the living room. He was visibly anxious and agitated as he described the dream. Defiance and opposition could fluctuate with anxiety and neediness from moment to moment; this was characteristic of Roger in the early months of therapy.

DIAGNOSTIC EVALUATION

I. Drive Assessment

The outstanding feature in Roger's presenting difficulties was his problem with aggression. He had a "hair-trigger" temper; he was exceedingly provocative and driven to prove his "toughness." The major source of his *aggressive drive difficulty* appeared to be at the phallic level of development. Early conflict emerged in his relationship to his father, who appeared as a major threat and "castrator" in Roger's perception. Roger appeared to react intensely and massively to early feelings of shame, humiliation, and smallness in relation to his father through extensive counterreaction. Thus, we see the massive defensive process. There was also some suggestion in this history that Roger was struggling with the impulses of cruelty and sadism, which are the aggressive drive components of the anal phase of development. His struggle with his father emerged during his toilet training at age 2½. An additional contribution to Roger's problems with aggression appeared to come from his endowment. He was described as a vigorous, energetic youngster from the beginning of his life, which suggests a strong constitutional inheritance of instinctual drives. This endowment could contribute to the aggressive conflict at all stages of development.

Despite Roger's impulsive behavior and his apparent unconcern for others in his attacks and disregard of rules, there was indication of a relatively higher level capacity for *object attachment*. During his early years, there was a good and "happy" interplay between parents and child. Roger also appeared to evidence the affect of guilt in the evaluation. He was greatly disturbed about his dream in which his mother's head was severed. It appeared that he felt guilty about the aggressive impulses directed at his mother that were manifested in the dream, although this was expressed as anxiety and agitation.

II. Ego Assessment

In many ways, Roger gave evidence of good ego functioning. Despite his behavior problems, he performed well at school academically and scored well in achievement tests. Basically, his ego functions were well developed—perception, memory, secondary process thinking, ability to abstract, and so forth. He also had a capacity to work at tasks (academic work) when his conflicts were not involved (e.g., his masculinity was not threatened). In the evaluation, however, there was some suggestion of ego weakness at times in relation to the strength of Roger's aggressive drives. He evidenced prominent accessibility to his aggression and found significant pleasure in his ability to intimidate peers (e.g., his classmates or siblings).

A very prominent feature in Roger's ego functioning was his response to internal conflicts with aggression. It appeared that Roger's phallic aggressive wishes promoted an anticipated anxiety response—that he would be attacked by a powerful authority (the castrator father). Roger appeared to have an enormous anxiety about castration during his development. He responded to this "threat" in a massive way. He used the defense mechanism of *identification with the aggressor* (or *turning passive into active*), and this defensive process became prominent, indeed, a central mechanism in Roger's life. In fact, at the time of the evaluation, Roger could be characterized by his antiauthority "macho" personality.

III. Superego Assessment

Problems in superego development seemed to fit the picture. In his development, Roger did experience the affects of shame, humiliation, and guilt that normally lead to the internalization (taking in) of the prohibitions of parents and other authorities. However, with Roger, the intensity of the feelings of shame, humiliation, and guilt led in another direction. The anxiety that these affects produced were so powerful that Roger had to defend against them. He identified with the threatening object (father) or the subject of the anxiety, and transformed himself into the threatening figure.

An important distinction between potentially psychopathic youngsters and neurotic characterologically disturbed children is whether the affects of shame and guilt are experienced at all, inasmuch as these affects are the "building blocks" of the conscience. Roger did experience these affects and then warded them off. One of the tasks of treatment was to help Roger experience them more readily, as discussed later in this chapter.

In the histories of youngsters like Roger, it is often difficult to reconstruct the early contributions of "nurture" and "nature." Whereas it seemed that Roger's instinctual endowment was a significant factor in his lifelong problems with aggression, the therapist had a lingering question about the capacity for parental empathy during these early years. These parents were clearly thoughtful, psychologically minded people at the time of the evaluation. However, in reviewing the toilet-training history, it seemed that they appeared *intent* on pushing for accomplishment despite their youngster's fears and intense reactions. Did this indicate some inability to assess their child's intense anxiety during this period? Such questions about parental contribution are often difficult to assess fully.

COURSE OF TREATMENT
Clinical Material: The Early Work

Roger was seen twice weekly for about 1½ years, and the course of the psychotherapy is described as it unfolded. During the early months of treatment, Roger highlighted his delinquent exploits in a highly pleasurable, excited, and heroic way. He thoroughly enjoyed the Lepke gang activities: They developed techniques as Peeping Toms; they had continuous rip-off plans for stealing from supermarkets, drug stores, and the like. They had a constant store of liquor, cigarettes, and pot, which they used in the group. They were involved in guarding the "turf" of the neighborhood, letting no alien young adolescents use the playground or ride bikes on the streets. They enjoyed attacking the rich. For example, throwing eggs at Cadillacs was great sport. Similar feats at school were described: Roger discussed his technique with spitballs, his protection of vulnerable girls against the older kids, and other such activities. His greatest disdain was for the frightened and weak boys. He noted, with contempt, that the "punks" and the "fags" that populated his school made him sick.

Roger appeared to have a number of motivations in providing this "heroic" material. He was pleased with the exhibitions of his exploits. He was also defiantly testing the therapist to see whether he would react with sanction and admonition. It was important for the therapist to maintain his relative neutrality. The gang attachment was part of an important pattern that the therapist and Roger would need to understand as the therapy went on.

Very occasionally there would be a session in marked contrast to the unfolding of these daily exploits. Roger would then be extremely agitated and markedly upset. For example, he was beset by thoughts that his father would have a car accident or die slowly of a heart ailment. He hated these thoughts and wanted therapy to get rid of them right now. He felt they would drive him crazy. He wanted to get away, to change schools, or move to another area where peace and tranquility could reign. The few occasions when guilt and anxiety reached consciousness created intolerable feeling states for him. The therapeutic task was to link this isolated misery with his more typical aggressive pleasure.

The therapist began to find occasions to make important connections. For example, the Lepke group, along with Roger, had been harassing an older couple in the neighborhood, a couple whom Roger really liked. He had delivered papers to them and cut their lawn. In their harassment, the gang would ring their doorbell and hide. The pleasure was watching these people sputter and get increasingly upset. Roger was responsive to the therapist's observation that he felt bad attacking these people, but a very important feeling drove him to join the harassment. *No matter what, Roger could not stand being accused of being a chicken. He would always act to wipe out any hint of babyish "punk-fag" feelings in himself.* This theme of wiping out any potential punk-fag feeling, no matter what the cost, became a very familiar refrain. He often reacted to his mother's concerns about his getting into trouble by yelling at her and breaking something. Again, he could slowly hear from the therapist that he felt her message was that he was a helpless little boy. His furious response was to show that there were no punk-fag feelings in him. His father's rules, on some occasions appropriate, always made him feel like a "little shit," and he was forced to act to wipe away that feeling. In fact, the therapist suggested again and again, his daily exploits were to quiet the inside "punk-fag-chicken" worry. On one occasion in this period, Roger acknowledged that when he was little, he was afraid he would be drafted into the army and killed in a war, and also afraid that his father was a member of the National Guard. He seemed to listen when the therapist responded that *all* little kids were frightened as they grew up when they looked at the big giant father, the father who was a mustache man, and that didn't really make them punk-fags.

Similar themes permeated the transference. He could get mad with his therapist whenever he wanted to, he declared. He did not have to listen to a shrink or anyone who told the lies that his therapist told him. Many sessions were filled with acts of defiance. He walked out of the office on occasion, or lit up a cigarette. Not only would he leave at will, but he also announced he would never return. The therapist became adept at spotting the need for the "tough Lepke gang" stance during the treatment hour. He told Roger that, internally, he needed to think about what made him need to be tough. Perhaps Roger was upset with the therapy because he had told the therapist about the army worry or because he was "complying" too much by coming to his sessions on time. These acts could carry a punk-fag valence for Roger and stimulate the intense affect of shame. Roger would then react with his characteristic defiance. The therapist began to articulate these dynamics within the hour, as it occurred in the transference. For example, on one occasion, after a series of good sessions, Roger spit repeatedly into the wastepaper basket and snarled for the first 20 minutes. The therapist commented that the "Lepke gang was certainly here today in full force." He thought that maybe they showed up because Roger had become worried about what was happening in treatment. Things had been going too well. If things continued this way, what would happen to his "bad temper"? The therapist wondered whether Roger worried that without his Lepke temper, he would feel weak and helpless. Roger translated, "You mean I might be worried that I'm going to become a pussy. Naw, I'm not worried about that," and he smiled broadly. Then Roger calmed down for the rest of the session.

Discussion

What techniques did the therapist employ in dealing with the character mode that Roger employed extensively? The therapist understood that Roger's driven "acting out" behavior was primarily based on conflict—he could not tolerate feeling small and helpless, and he was driven to erase that internal image.

The concept of *defense analysis*—repeated, repetitious interventions aimed at working through maladaptive behaviors that are pervasive resistances—is the key intervention with children with character pathology. Some of Wilhelm Reich's early work on character analysis (1963) is especially applicable. If we look closely at the preceding clinical material, we can delineate a series of interventions in the process of *defense analysis* with Roger. This process involves four steps: (1) making the particular behavior (character trait) explicit to the patient's ego; (2) making the ego-syntonic behavior (character trait) somewhat more alien to the patient; (3) making the underlying motivation for the behavior conscious to the patient; (4) making these motivations, formerly frightening, acceptable to the patient.

Initially the therapist defined Roger's behavior. The therapist *confronted* and *clarified* the action in question: "Roger often needs to act tough"; "Roger needs to defy adults, break rules at home and school"; "Roger needs to prove he is as tough as the older kids." Roger's general stance and the associated behaviors were explicitly brought to his attention. This quality was defined as Roger's "tough Lepke-gang stance" and became a metaphor in the treatment hour.

A major early goal in the work with Roger was to make some of this explicit behavior *ego-alien*, though it had previously given him great pleasure. Feelings of unpleasure that Roger experienced (loss of self-esteem, guilt, loss of parental love) were affects that emerged but were *split off* from Roger's acts and not seen as connected. It was enormously helpful to clearly link some of the dreadful internal consequences that he experienced with Roger's daily behavior. Thus, the therapist clarified that Roger's provocation (with the Lepke gang) of the older neighborhood couple *did* make him feel very guilty. He felt bad later and uneasy with himself. Similarly, the anxiety dreams about his father's health often emerged after Roger had given his father a very hard time. He seemed to worry that his troubling behavior with his father could seriously affect the older man and hated himself for the problems he was causing. Similarly, he often seemed to be very upset after a big blowup with his mother. The internal and hidden cost of his driven exploits become clearer to Roger and tarnished the sense of pure pleasure with the action-macho image.

The prominent and repeated *interpretations* were the therapist's comments that Roger's tough behavior pushed away the *normal* helpless internal affects of childhood. As noted earlier, the process of "identification with the aggressor" warded off a sense of weakness and helplessness, which had induced shame and humiliation. Slowly verbalizing the self-images that Roger feared (the punk–fag fears) and providing an acceptable developmental context for them were critical elements of the treatment process. Any command or request by parent, teacher, or therapist was seen by Roger as an attack on his self-esteem, an attempt to bring him to his knees. These "humiliations" made him need to act defiantly quickly. Slowly, Roger came to accept that although he could feel small (be given an assignment by a teacher or a chore by his father), the "small" feeling was typical for all children and young boys. He, however, tended to experience these requests as an enormous put-downs and reacted to them as major slights. In order to *work through* Roger's defensive overreaction, this interpretive theme was repeated very often in the course of the work. This was particularly effective in the transference—when Roger became tough in the session, the therapist searched for the material of the hour (or the previous hour) that could have provoked a sense of humiliation.

Why is the therapist primarily limited to *defense analysis*? Much of the focus of the work is intended to deal with extensive variations of a particular form of maladaptive behavior. Because Roger used this central defense pervasively, repeated intervention became necessary. In addition, children with character pathology do not tolerate extensive reconstruction of the past history that originally fostered the need for the pervasive defensive reaction. One can speculate that the reason Roger's phallic and oedipal struggle with the "castrating" father became so intense was that his underlying dependency needs and feminine wishes were particularly prominent factors in his development. One may also speculate that for children like Roger, the early experiences of childhood would be even more beset by intense anxiety than for neurotic children, inasmuch as they resort to massive defensive reactions. Intense anxiety states interfere with the development of cognitive functioning and growing verbal and symbolic capacity. These factors can make it more difficult for a reconstructive process to take place in children with character pathology.

Clinical Material: The Later Work

The work with Roger during the first year did not only involve identifying his need to act to ward off helpless affects. He also had many difficulties just containing stored-up rage. The therapist witnessed an already familiar pattern, an outbreak of rage and, later, apparently unconnected self-loathing. For example, on one occasion, the whole family attended a piano recital by Roger's sister, who was an accomplished musician. Later, in the celebration at a restaurant, Roger had made an incredible scene, defiantly yelling at a minor request by his father. He ended by screaming, "I hate families," and the L family was forced to leave the restaurant abruptly. When the therapist discussed the event with Roger (the therapist had received the "news of the week in review" from the parents), Roger focused on his father's rotten behavior. However, his characteristic smile of pleasure emerged when the therapist attempted to reconstruct his feelings of the afternoon: how much he must have hated his sister, his wish that she would make a mistake during the concert and screw up, and how good it felt to finally ruin her day and get all his angry feelings out. The therapist predicted that he would later have a strong "black sheep" feeling. Roger responded immediately by talking of a dream he had recently had, about a dog the family had onced owned. In the dream the dog had "pissed and shit" all over the house and was taken by the collar to the Humane Society by his father. It was clear Roger felt that he was the incorrigible dog who would be thrown out of the family and killed. The themes of his constant daily rage with those close-knit family members, his intense pleasure at upsetting them, his strong feelings of being the outsider, became very familiar ideas.

Roger began to speak more of his internal life. He talked about stories and books he had read. Prominent were the stories of a white boy raised by Indians, and a child who lost his parents in World War II and survived in a concentration camp. When his feelings of being the abandoned orphan were discussed, Roger told his therapist of his conviction that he was really adopted and that he had often searched the house for his "papers." He came to identify these upsetting "black sheep" feelings and also began to realize that his daily rage *did* make people treat him differently in the family. Roger developed an increasing awareness that his own behavior and the parental counterreactions promoted his sense of being different, adopted, rejected. With this material, after a year of work, Roger's behavior began to change. He began working with his father, doing heavy "manly" construction work on the house, and redesigning furniture for his room. His father found him an energetic and amazing worker.

During the last 6 months of therapy, there were many behavior fluctuations in a good–bad Roger, with increasing periods of control. He still had numerous problems on the school playground and smilingly told his therapist he had a magnet in his pocket that attracted fights. The therapist noted that it was hard for him to tolerate the feelings (the identity) of being good. The therapist coined the phrase, "A fight during the day keeps the punk feelings away." A sudden disruptive episode with a teacher he was beginning to like was respresentative. Mrs. G was a teacher of German extraction, and one day he came to salute her with "Sieg heil" in the classroom and answer all questions with "Ja wohl." It slowly became clear that he had become increasingly fond of her, was being used by her as a class monitor, and that he was overwhelmed with a "goody-two-shoes" feeling. His reaction was to disrupt the needy, caring, and tender identity.

Roger increasingly discussed feelings that made him embarrassed. He had some current worries. He was still afraid of the army and was relieved that there was no draft any longer. At times he had bad dreams. After seeing *Jaws* (the movie), he was beset by shark dreams. He recalled more childhood night fears of a white hand trying to choke him or pirates who cut off limbs with a sword. Attempts to move into underlying sexual anxieties and masturbation were met with intense resistance. For example, when the therapist brought up the idea that often guys' concerns about damaged limbs had to do with their fears of touching themselves, Roger could not work with that kind of internal material. But Roger's daily self-observation increased. He reported potential "dares" that the former (before treatment) Roger would get involved in. For example, in the past he often would break up some football play of older boys, intercept the pass, and run off. Although he had similar urges, he now refrained. He knew the urge was just to prove that he was not scared and that became a stupid idea because he would always get beaten up.

With Roger's sustained good functioning, there was pressure from him and parents to stop treatment. At termination, it was suggested that there might be flare-ups in the future and stated that the therapist would be available for any crisis work.

Discussion

In the preceding treatment material, there was an important shift in the course of the work. Roger himself actively identified his provocative–defiant patterns and self-observed the process. For example, he commented that he had been tempted to provoke the older kids on the schoolyard but refrained. The patterns became more ego-alien because he was much more aware of the "black sheep" consequences (his own punitive superego). However, when the therapist pointed out his fears of tender, caring feelings (e.g., toward the teacher) that promoted acting out, Roger could tolerate limited only exploration of the threat of his "soft" feelings.

In the later stages of treatment, Roger could tolerate the therapist's descriptions and verbalizations of his primitive rage and destructiveness. For example, the therapist reconstructed the proud recital day—Roger's hatred of his sister, his wish that she would err during her performance, and his desire to ruin the celebration at the restaurant. The therapist added a human dynamic—Roger had these feelings because he was jealous, and these are common sibling experiences. The purpose of verbalizing these constructions and providing a context for them was to modify Roger's own unduly harsh internal reactions to these destructive wishes.

There are some important counterreactive tendencies and issues within the therapist that typically emerge when he or she is confronted with the sustained defiance and provocative behaviors of such youngsters. What are the internal reactions of the therapist to having smoke blown in his or her face, having "asshole" written on all available newsprint, and having the theme of uselessness of therapy constantly elaborated on? Three major counterreactions are stimulated within the therapy with children like Roger. A common reaction is rage, which is often handled by expression in some direct or subtle way within the treatment or by suppression of these "unacceptable" feelings. For example, with a reaction fueled by the natural anger these patients evoke, it is not uncommon to make a direct, forceful intervention. On one occasion, the therapist was describing how isolated Roger was from his peers because of his behavior. He became aware that in his description of the rejection Roger was experiencing, he was "twisting the knife" so that Roger could fully experience the pain. On self-examination, the motive for this "intervention" was revenge.

Another major reaction is a subtle admiration for these young-sters who, on the surface, appear as though they are afraid of noth-ing. Partly, the therapist is impressed with their evident "masculin-ity." A third typical counterreaction is fatigue as a reaction to the provocation coupled with a desire to shut off the search for an empathic response. The transactional dynamic is that the defiant child presses the therapist to repeat the past relationships—provocation of the adult authority and angry counterreaction. The feelings of having extended oneself, "gone the extra mile" for the youngster, are often intense internal reactions that can lead to a ces-sation of the therapeutic process. The therapist's understanding of the patient's internal dynamics, therefore, is vital for his dealing with the counterreactive trends. For instance, when Roger walked out of the treatment office telling the therapist he had better things to do, it became clear that he was trying to make the therapist feel small and helpless. Something was happening currently that had induced these unacceptable feelings (smallness, helplessness) within Roger, and Roger was attempting to reverse the situation in his characteristic way. The therapist could then use this information (Roger's attempt to externalize his feelings of helplessness) to understand Roger's cur-rent struggle. Such mechanisms are common transference paradigms with these youngsters.

The difficulty a therapist typically has in sustaining his or her empathic capacity with the intensely defiant child patient brings us to some of the diagnostic considerations discussed earlier. I have dis-cussed some of the "nature" and "nurture" contributions to the pa-thology of these children. Children like Roger are typically described as "intense," "active," and "driven" from birth, and this speaks to the heightened instinctual endowment we often find in these young-sters. They also approach each developmental task intensely. Thus, when Roger struggled with the developmental issues of autonomy and limits, he appeared vigorous and defiant (rather than frightened and terrified at times) to his parents. Although his parents reacted somewhat with force (e.g., in toilet training) rather than understand-ing, can we say there was a major failure of parental empathy that caused the developmental interference in Roger's growth? In my ex-perience with youngsters like Roger, it is clear that they often need unusually tolerant and empathic parents to fare well in development, and typically adequate parents often do badly with these children who need more.

SUMMARY

In summation, there are a number of important similarities, differences, and limits in the treatment of children with character pathology as compared with those with neurosis. The work with many children with character problems is a form of insight-oriented, uncovering treatment. Essentially, in the work with Roger, the therapist helped him to gain insight into the unconscious motivation of his character pattern. In this sense, the psychotherapy was "uncovering" and "interpretive" (bringing into consciousness what has been unconscious), as with neurotic children. However, there are many differences. In work with character pathology, insight is primarily limited to *defense analysis*, and there is a minimum of *content analysis* (exploring the underlying wishes and fantasies and placing them in a historical context). In the treatment process with Fred, the neurotic youngster (Chapter 6), there was a good deal of treatment of the defenses (resistances) when his mechanisms of intellectualization, isolation, etc., were analyzed. In addition, however, Fred engaged in major content analysis and more fully explored the roots of his aggression, dependency wishes, and sexual and masochistic longings, using memories and dreams that reconstructed the past. This fuller exploration is much less available in work with children with character pathology.

BIBLIOGRAPHY

Abend, S. (1983). Theory of character. *Journal of the American Psychoanalytic Association* 31:211–224.

Fissler, K. (1948). Ego-psychological implication of the psychoanalytic treatment of delinquents. *Psychoanalytic Study of the Child* 5:97–121.

Fenichel, O. (1945). *The Psychoanalytic Theory of Neurosis*. New York: W. W. Norton.

Feranczi, S. (1942). Gulliver fantasies. *International Journal of Psychoanalysis* 23:221–228.

Freud, A. (1946). *The Ego and Mechanisms of Defense*. New York: International Universities Press.

Freud, S. (1937). *Analysis Terminable and Interminable* (Standard Ed., Vol. 23). London: Hogarth Press.

Johnson, A. M., & Szurek, S. A. (1952). The genesis of the antisocial acting out in children and adults. *The Psychoanalytic Quarterly* 21:323–343.

Michaels, J., & Stiver, I. (1965). The impulsive psychopathic character according to the diagnostic profile. *Psychoanalytic Study of the Child* 20:124–141.

Redl, F., & Wineman, D. (1951). *Children Who Hate*. Glencoe, IL: Free Press.

Reich, W. (1963). *Character Analysis*. New York: Noonday Press.

Rexford, E. N. (1952). A developmental concept of the problems of acting out. *Journal of the American Academy of Child Psychiatry* 2:6–21.

Rexford, E. N. (1959). Antisocial young children and their families. In: L. Jessner & F. Pavenstead (Eds.), *Dynamic Psychopathology in Childhood* (pp. 186–220). New York: Grune & Stratton.

Stein, M. (1969). The problem of character theory. *Journal of the American Psychoanalytic Association* 17:675–701.

8

~

Treatment of
the Borderline Child

In this chapter and the next, the focus is on the treatment of children with borderline and narcissistic disturbances. The pathologies represent the more severe psychopathologies of childhood, and they tend to be viewed as disturbances centering in early object development (the early relationship with the caregiving adult). Therefore, in order to understand the treatment strategy with these youngsters, it is helpful to review some early object relations theory so that the therapist can have a conceptual framework of this period of development.

In addition, the processes of treatment with these disturbances are described. With the severe pathologies, treatment techniques tend to be "supportive," rather than "uncovering" like those employed with the neurotic child. When the patient is more fragile, it is generally disruptive to functioning to "uncover" the instinctual life. The supportive techniques are aimed at "shoring up" or building the ego. This is done by stabilizing and fostering the development of ego functions (e.g., reality testing) or the specific ego defenses.

Therefore, as the case of a borderline child is examined in this chapter, there are two major themes: (1) understanding this youngster's pathology in light of problems in early object attachment and separation and (2) examining the ego-building and supportive techniques the therapist can employ in dealing with the borderline patient.

A REVIEW OF EARLY OBJECT RELATIONS THEORY: THE DEVELOPMENTAL CONTEXT FOR BORDERLINE AND NARCISSISTIC DISTURBANCES

The pioneering work of Margaret Mahler (1952, 1968) (elaborated by Furer; Settledge [1977]; and Pine [1974]) focused on the early phases of development of the infant, particularly in relation to the progression of attachment and separation from the object (caregiving individual). The object relations theory (the course of attachment and separation from the caregiver in the first few years of life) that has emerged has a similar structure to drive theory (course of the sexual and aggressive drive). In drive theory, there is a progression through natural phases of development (oral, anal, phallic, oedipal, latency, adolescence) for the child to traverse. For the best outcome in development, the child needs to move successfully through conflicts at each specific phase of development. Arrest or fixation (a lack of progression of the sexual or aggressive drive) in any phase can create the basis for pathology in adulthood. For example, severe problems in the normal oral phase can be the basis for eating disorders in adolescence and adulthood (for example, bulimia, anorexia, obesity). Problems at the oral phase can produce a fixation, expressed in later life through a variety of symptoms or behaviors. For example, having a very depressed and absent mother as an infant can produce an anxiety about starvation. This "oral anxiety" can then become a preoccupation throughout life, a fixation at the oral level, because of the intensity of the early problem. In early life, a youngster may attempt to deal with this difficulty by overeating. Later, any anxiety could produce the "symptom" of overeating. We would then see the legacy of the early fixation in this individual's adult psychopathology expressed in obesity or an ever-present anxiety or preoccupation with food.

In a similar way, Mahler (1952, 1968) outlined the process (phases) of early attachment and separation that the infant and young child must progress through. Arrest or fixation along this continuum of development provides the legacy for the severe developmental pathologies of childhood.

The following is a condensed summary of this progression. In the early weeks of development up until 2 months of age, all infants experience the "normal autistic" phase wherein they are, as yet, un-

attached to the object (mother). At this point, the infant has no connection to the object, and the beginning connection becomes stimulated by the care and ministrations of the caregiver. The normal
autistic phase is seen by Mahler as an objectless phase.*

In normal development, in accordance with the pleasure principle (through the adequate care, feeding, playing, with the child, etc.,
that are experienced as pleasurable to the child), the child "attaches"
to the parent figure. The nature of that early normal attachment is a
symbiotic one, whereby the infant cannot distinguish himself from
the object. This second early phase of object development is called
the "phase of primary narcissism" (Freud, 1914) or the period of
"symbiotic union" (Mahler, 1968). This normal phase has a number
of characteristics. During this phase, (1) the child cannot distinguish
between self and other, (2) he experiences a growing sense of omnipotence and magic gratification, and (3) all good experiences are part
of the emerging self, whereas bad experiences are expelled outside
the self.

In these early months the child cannot distinguish the physical
boundaries between himself and his mother. For example, by 9 to 10
months, he may be aware of the word "nosey" and know which part
of the body this refers to. However, it is not until a number of
months later that he can distinguish between "his nosey" and
"Mommy's nosey." At the phase of symbiotic union, there is a natural fusion of the child's and the caretaker's physical boundaries.

The child also experiences omnipotence and a sense of magic
gratification at this stage of development. Most mothers are very sensitive to their babies' needs and have learned their babies' signals and
cries. They can often distinguish between the hungry, the need-to-be-
changed, and the I-want-to-be-held signals. The young child experiences these ministrations and gratifications of needs as magic, and he
experiences an early sense of omnipotence (if I have a need, it will be
met).

The world surrounding the young child is conceived as "all pleasurable," and he expels any frustration to the "outside" or the
nonself. We speak of this period as a time when normal "splitting"

---

*In the more recent infant developmental literature, researchers describe very early active
connection to the environment and objects. For further information, the reader is referred
to Stern and Sander (1980).

occurs, where the "good" world is central to the self, and the "bad" world is protruded to the outside. Inasmuch as the *phase of primary narcissism* or *symbiotic union* is part of the normal experience of development, there is a natural legacy for all individuals to recreate this early Garden of Eden, where there is no frustration and endless gratification exists. For example, one of the facets of the "perfect vacation"—lying on a beach surrounded by the warm sun and sand, no daily cares, perfect meals, and so on—seems to embody a return to the characteristics of the period of primary narcissism.

If major problems occur in this phase of development (because of internal organic factors within the child or major problems in the environment), there can be an arrest or fixation in this symbiotic phase. An early form of childhood psychosis is the "symbiotic–psychotic child" (Mahler, 1968), one of the severe developmental psychopathologies. These children have marked disturbances in their body boundaries. For example, one such child patient of mine feared that his facial characteristics might change. He was afraid to look into a mirror because his face could turn into the face of his mother. Another child was afraid to go into the water because he could not see his legs. He feared these extremities would cease to exist if they weren't in sight. There was no sense of solidity to his physical self. These children often have similar problems with boundaries outside the body, physical boundaries in space and size. They fear that buildings can disappear or rooms can suddenly change. There is often no solidness to the world at large for such children. These fears reflect difficulties in fusion, characteristic of the period of symbiotic union. The pathology of these children is severe and falls into the realm of childhood psychosis. With the perceptional distortions they develop, there are marked difficulties in the function of reality testing (the ability to know the difference between an internal and external perception or thought). It is primarily the function of reality testing that distinguishes the psychotic from the nonpsychotic individual.

Slowly, beginning in the latter part of the first year, the child normally progresses from the symbiotic phase to the period of separation–individuation. This encompasses a number of steps or subphases (hatching, practicing, rapprochement, libidinal object constancy) that are achieved by the end of the third year. In this process, the child moves from the magic world to reality and from the normal narcissistic stage to a shared world with objects (parents, siblings, and peers). There are a number of tasks the young child must achieve to make this effective transition into reality: (1) a gradual giving up of the sense of omnipotence, (2) the ability to separate self from object, as well as (3) the capacity to synthesize the "good" and "bad" aspects of the object and the self. Much of the impetus for separation–individuation comes from the child's ability to locomote (crawling, standing, walking) and the enormous pleasures derived from the sense of mastery in self-achievement through action in reality. For example, when a toddler sees a ball across the room that he desires, and he crawls or walks to get it himself, he experiences an internal pleasure of accomplishment by his own action. This internal pleasure of the autonomous self grows and becomes the force for separation from the object and fosters the sense of individuation.

During the past 10 years, infant observers and researchers have modified some of Mahler's conceptions, particularly of the earliest infant phases. Most researchers now question the existence of a "normal autistic" phase and indicate that the infant is social and active from birth. They see the initial period from birth to 2 months of life as a phase of normal emergence or awakenings rather than an objectless one (Stern, 1985).

Similarly, in the period of 2 to 7 months, the period of "symbiotic union" prior to separation–individuation, there are also modifications. The processes of fusion of self and other as well as the emergence of the individual self are definitely observed in early childhood. However, rather than distinct phases following each other, these processes are seen as occurring and unfolding simultaneously from the early months. Whatever the timetable, the processes of symbiosis and separation–individuation do occur.

Early interferences in the separation–individuation process (constitutional factors, severe illness in childhood, major problems in parent–child relationship) can affect this progression and lay the foundation for further severe pathology in childhood. Problems in the separation–individuation phase can be the breeding ground for "borderline" and "narcissistic" disturbances (Chethik & Fast, 1970; Chethik, 1979; Settledge, 1977; Meissner, 1978). Borderline pathology reflects a partial transition out of the process of symbiotic union. The borderline child has become able to separate self from other, and he therefore has no problems with body boundaries or with the boundaries in reality. He does not exhibit the psychotic processes evident in the symbiotic child, according to many authors. However, he fails in several other tasks. The borderline child retains "splitting," and objects and self-representations must be divided into "good" and "bad." In addition, some aspects of magic and omnipotence are also maintained.

It is helpful to understand the meaning of "splitting" more fully. Splitting is a normal mechanism in early childhood. The young child naturally pushes away any images of the angry mother (she is not my mother; she is someone else), and he retains a feeling of safety with only positive images of the mother. This is reflected in children's fascination with fairy tales, tales young children love because they reflect their internal struggles. The good fairy godmother is the symbol for the all-giving mother who provides everything, whereas the evil wicked witch or the wicked stepmother (*Cinderella, Hansel and Gretel*) is the repository of all of the frustration and projected punishments by the object. The world is divided into good and evil. The young child splits the maternal images into these extremes. During separation–individuation, a task for the growing youngster is to become increasingly able to put together these diverse images of mother and to retain some aspects of both. The images of the angry mother or the grouchy mother must become part of the overall caregiver who is the provider depended on. The ability to achieve this reality view of the object depends, in part, on the quality of frustration by the object—how he or she disciplines, withholds, and demands—as well as on the subject's own internal equipment. The borderline child *fails* to accomplish this developmental task. Clearly, the vast majority of children achieve this step.

With this background, we can now follow the presentation and the treatment process of a borderline youngster, Matthew, a 10-year-old in a residential treatment center.

MATTHEW: PRESENTING PICTURE, HISTORY, AND DIAGNOSTIC THOUGHTS

Matthew was placed at Sagebrook treatment center because of chronic problems that made him unable to function in the community. Essentially, in the classroom he had been seen as "strange" and "always in his own world." He muttered sounds, seemed unable to learn (he had spent years in the special education program), and rarely spoke to the teacher. At times, without any apparent provocation or predictability, he had become agitated, terrified, and had acted impulsively, totally disrupting the classroom. On these occasions, he had been very hard to contain.

Similarly at home, he withdrew into the "safety" of his room and had fought any excursions outside the house. His growing isolation and withdrawal had concerned his parents increasingly.

In the residential center, a similar picture emerged in the first few months after placement. Matthew was quickly nicknamed "Cartoon Boy" by the other children in the cottage. Each day would find him totally engrossed in himself in a corner of his room, producing his shows and cartoons. A cartoon was introduced by the appropriate Looney Tunes melody; one heard the sounds of the chase, the scuffling, the ultimate victory of his characters, and the cartoon was clearly over when the last few fading bars of the introductory melody were repeated. His hero, Popeye, was represented by a little plastic toy figure, who vigorously fought off pursuing monsters and attacking tornadoes with great animation. When the demands of the day interrupted Matthew's cartooning—for example, when he was called to lunch—he managed to announce "intermission" and very tentatively and fearfully proceeded to join his cottage mates in the dining room.

During his early years, Matthew seemed to evidence a constitutional vulnerability. His mother, a wholesome woman who cared very adequately for two other siblings, described a nightmare-like first year of development for this child. At first Matthew had been unable to suck. He had cried constantly during the day. Often his distress reached screaming intensity without any evident source of irritation or frustration. His parents finally found that the only way to soothe him was to drive him endlessly in the family car. Even when he slept, Matthew was obviously fussy and troubled.

Throughout the first year, Matthew was tense and stiff when held in his mother's arms. He arched his back away from her, and she found herself unable to calm him. Mrs. M had trouble with feeding. As the year progressed, Matthew refused to chew and would not take liquids other than milk and cocoa.

At age 4, his mother described him as an "albatross around her neck." She could not limit him. At the supermarket he ran throughout the store pulling items off the shelves and jumping and climbing over counters. The mother was unable to visit with anyone when accompanied by Matthew, because he was restless and needed constant supervision.

At times, Matthew yelled and screamed in a very infantile way, and tantrums, produced by very minor frustrations, were an everyday affair. With Matthew present, the mother found it very difficult to share her attention. He seemed jealous and interfered with her when she was on the telephone. Matthew also refused to do anything for himself—he refused to try to unbutton his jacket and waited for Mother to take off his hat and coat.

In contrast to his usual wildness and distractability, within the limits of his familiar room Matthew could play for hours. He could sit and listen to his records over and over again and play with a group of plastic soldiers for long periods of time. However, his mother experienced an uneasy feeling because at these times, in the course of this play, Matthew would often let out a peculiar shriek for no apparent reason. His mother also noted some of Matthew's occasional efforts to restrain himself. He doubled up his fists and made squeezing noises as if to keep himself from breaking things.

Matthew presented evidence of a longstanding developmental disorder. In their histories, borderline children typically show major disruption in the first year of life. Matthew's history revealed early disturbing feeding experiences and major problems with the ability to be soothed and gratified by objects. Throughout his childhood, Matthew showed profound problems in three major areas of development: drive development, ego development, and object relations development.

DIAGNOSTIC EVALUATION

I. Drive Assessment

Matthew, like many borderline children, struggled in an attempt to deal with primitive pregenital aggression (Kernberg, 1975). In normal development, when a child can give up the early mechanism of "splitting" into good and evil, it is implict that the "evil" and aggressive world is less frightening. For example, the images of the angry or grouchy mother can become part of the good mother he depends on, because the angry mother is not so frightening. This is not true for the borderline child. The "bad" outside world continues to retain the early primitive terror. This terror continues to plague the borderline youngster as he develops.

Matthew attempted to handle this frightening world through his "cartoon" fantasy life. This appeared to serve two functions: he withdrew from the real, "frightening" world into his own fantasy life, and within the fantasy world he sought to master the dangers. His fantasy life was filled with aggressive monsters and tornadoes, a representation of the split-off bad world of the narcissistic phase of development. He magically mastered the danger by becoming Popeye, super-strong when he swallowed the can of spinach, to overcome every adversary. He retained the magic solutions typical of the narcissistic period of life. Thus, borderline children struggle continuously with primitive aggression and do not achieve the neutralization (dilution) of the aggressive drive seen in normal development.

II. Ego Assessment

Matthew's presentation and history evidenced the generalized weak ego functioning that is commonly associated with many borderline children. It is generally the task of the ego in normal development to handle and negotiate the "threats" to the self that come from either internal or external sources. For example, by age 4, the normal child is expected to adapt to a new nursery school situation and function and learn therein, despite being separated from the mother. The young child's ego can typically cope with the potential threats of this new environment. Bigger or aggressive children will not be overwhelming, because the average child can place trust in the new mother substitutes in the school.

Most borderline children do not have the ego capacity to adapt to new surroundings. At age 4, Matthew was constantly overwhelmed by a feared threat in any new surround. He became restless, agitated, driven, and out of control in the supermarket, even in the presence of his mother. All new stimuli terrified him, and he felt safe only in the close confines of his room. He appeared to be constantly traumatized and had no effective adaptive or defensive system to negotiate the daily environment. He had built a wall of isolation and fantasy (cartoon world) that increasingly separated him physically from the world. He clung to outside objects (mother) to manage him, to function as an auxiliary ego, and to provide a source of safety.

Object Relations Assessment

Borderline children typically relate to objects on a "need-gratifying" basis, which is an early form of object tie associated with the narcissistic or symbiotic processes of development. The "all-good" object will fulfill all wishes, and the helpless child is totally dependent on the object for survival. This form of relationship is retained by the borderline youngster often throughout childhood, and forms of this interaction are retained by the borderline adult.

Throughout Matthew's history, his mother was forced to serve as his need gratifier. She had to provide constant attention, and even the telephone (taking attention away from Matthew) was perceived as a threat. Matthew was anxious about any independent step he would need to take as it would separate him from his mother. Therefore, his mother had to button his jacket, for example, well beyond the time he could physically cope with this skill. Borderline children often experience panic and terror with separation from the "object" who keeps them safe, and they are also coersive with the object. They demand attention because they fear that if the object shows independence, the object can leave them.

Often these children will also withdraw from objects because of the perceived pain and lack of gratification in the real world and real attachments. They people their fantasy life with the omnipotent, protective, need-satisfying objects they seek. For Matthew, Popeye was a protector with his magic strength. The perceived frustrations of the real objects pushed Matthew to develop an extensive fantasy world and to develop a schizoid-like posture by his withdrawal into a narcissistic fantasy life (the cartoon world). This is a typical solution for many borderline children.

Matthew was seen initially more than 10 years ago. He had had a number of neurological workups, including an electroencephalogram (EEG) and a neurological exam. There was no overt evidence of brain damage. In recent years, however, there has been more extensive development of diagnostic tools to pick up subtle brain malfunctions. A youngster like Matthew would also currently receive medication trials to augment psychotherapy, because effective drugs have been developed to help these youngsters. Medication would be used in conjunction with hospitalization (residential treatment) and psychotherapy.

We now focus on the typical psychological treatment problems the therapist faces in work with the borderline child and the techniques and interventions he or she is often called on to employ. These are illustrated by the treatment of Matthew:

1. The emergence of the narcissistic fantasy life of the patient
2. The problem of the lack of repression

3. The coersive quality of the object tie
4. The problems of poor structuralization

COURSE OF TREATMENT

Dealing with the Narcissistic Fantasy Life

Clinical Material

When treatment began, Matthew sat in the far corner of the therapist's office with his back to the therapist. Only roars, grimaces, and screams were emitted as the course of his imagined cartoon progressed. Matthew was clearly terrified of the therapist. He surrounded himself with his cartoons, and there was no recognition that the therapist existed for many weeks. The therapist, from his own growing extensive knowledge of cartoons from Saturday morning TV watching, began identifying the specific characters from across the room. The therapist wrote up a movie program of each session. All the varied cartoons were listed in order of presentation, and because Matthew had a vast variety of characters, he would pack in as many as 20 cartoons in the 50-minute hour. Matthew left the corner of the room and, responding to the therapist's interest, unfolded the program on the therapist's desk. He corrected the therapist's titles and named each cartoon. They collected the programs in a special drawer, and Matthew took pleasure in reading the old programs as well as developing new ones. This introduction took a period of 4 months.

After this long period, Matthew decided on a change—he would include some full-length features in his movie house. He particularly wanted to add an adventure serial, and it became highly desired that the therapist have a prominent role. In the film, the therapist was the big protector, as he and the little boy took on very frightening elements. They faced spooky and haunted houses together, high winds and hurricanes, bad doctors who gave terrible shots. Matthew produced a long film called "World War II." The therapist (directed by Matthew) saved Matthew from torpedoed boats, artillery fire, and strafing fighter planes.

After about 8 months of work, the therapist introduced his own variation into the program, the idea of a documentary. Any good movie house must have a documentary, he proclaimed. He insisted that this documentary contain the essential element of a documentary—it had to reflect and record a true event. Although Matthew eagerly agreed at first, he subtly fought and tested out the new rule. For example, Matthew at first brought in documentary weather reports. On a lovely spring day he described the deep snow, slippery walking conditions, and so forth. Or he described the different fish he saw on a visit to the aquarium, but added wings to the fish and made them fly. The therapist pounded on the desk, noting that this was a violation of the documentary idea, and the weather and fish reports were not accepted until changed.

Documentary "true" talks assumed a more prominent role in the sessions. They began to reflect real affect. Matthew introduced the documentaries entitled "Homesick," "Home Sweet Home," "Learning about Sagebrook," and the like. Matthew described his feelings of loss of home, his present terror, and his questions about the institution.

In his documentaries about Sagebrook, an observing ego began to grow, and some aspects of a therapeutic alliance (rather than the earlier omnipotent protecting relationship) emerged. As "Cartoon Boy" Matthew felt he did not have any friends in the cottage; he felt very lonely, and he wanted boys to like him. Matthew noted that he hated the name "Cartoon Boy," and he made his own special contract with the therapist that the cartoons would eventually be stopped. He even fixed a specific date several months hence. Matthew then brought a new film—a "Sports Reel"—into the sessions, in which he vividly became a great baseball hero and football giant. The therapist interpreted that he had a great wish to be liked and to play with the other boys and develop his skills. Changes in Matthew's sessions were reflected in his daily life. He fought his cartooning and narrowed the cartoon time spent each day in his room. He practiced baseball and football with the child care worker he felt close to, and he began to participate in cottage meetings.

Discussion

The work within the psychotherapy reflected only a small part of the treatment work at the time. Matthew's beginning turn toward reality and self-observation could not have occurred without a concurrent and very active "milieu therapy" (Bettleheim, 1971). To use Nosphitz's (1971) term, the child with massive ego weakness must be "englobed" by treatment—not 1 hour three times per week, but consistently for many hours each day. The residential treatment center or hospital setting provides an opportunity to utilize fully this enveloping form of therapy. The therapist needs to work closely with the others in the milieu to help them understand the internal life of the child so that a strategy can be devised to deal with the child's underlying problems.

Matthew was frightened by his own destructive potential and

that of the environment. In cartoons, the characters he identified with met and mastered each projected danger. His withdrawal separated him from the unpleasant and frightening reality as his attention centered on his fantasy life. He denied his internal helplessness through magical omnipotent means: Popeye, when overwhelmed by danger, always had available a can of spinach that provided the strength to cope with all threats. For Matthew, cartoons warded off the unpredictable reality.

The function, then, of the early milieu work was to make the reality predictable and concrete. With help from the therapist, an outer stabilization and structure was provided in Matthew's daily life. The child care staff actively preplanned with Matthew what was in store for each day. His schedule was described, at first, on almost an hourly basis; he was helped to learn which staff members went off duty, and who came on to work. Any change in routine, or expectation of visitors, or furniture alteration, whenever possible, was discussed with Matthew beforehand. As Matthew had earlier listed his cartoon schedule, he now wrote out the daily cottage schedule, and his ability to anticipate events and changes allowed him slowly to become a fringe member. Only with this consistent milieu backdrop, actively initiated and supported by the therapist, could the work and progress in the psychotherapy continue. This process of interpreting the underlying anxieties to those within the milieu, and creating a structure to counter these fears, is an essential part of the work with many borderline children.

In helping Matthew work toward reality *within* the psychotherapy, it was also initially critical to understand the function of his fantasy world. As noted earlier, Matthew was struggling with "split-off" terrors he was unable to integrate. He attempted to cope with the world utilizing the mechanisms (magic, omnipotence) of the small child during the narcissistic stage of development. The therapist slowly *joined* his world by identifying and explicating his "cartoon shows." Over a period of time, they collected more than 100 cartoon show programs. Attempting to gain entry to the fantasy life and being admitted by the borderline child is often a necessary and critical initial step in the treatment process. The fantasy life of the child is often the most highly invested (cathected) area in the child's psychic existence, and the initial task of the therapist is to become an important part of that internal life.

Matthew, deriving increasing pleasure from this growing *mutual* movie production, decided to expand and include the therapist in full-length feature serials as well. He used the therapist in these productions as a narcissistic, need-satisfying protector. In his adventures Matthew had the therapist rescue the little boy from sharks, tornadoes, and bad doctors. This had a similar dynamic as the cartoon world, as together they fought the split-off evil world, but Matthew was establishing a strong libidinal (loving) tie to the therapist.

As their relationship grew, the therapist began to slowly demand that Matthew incorporate the real world. He noted that whereas every movie house has cartoons and full-length features, the really good theaters also had documentaries. The therapist began to function like a facilitating parent who helps his frightened toddler to integrate aspects of the "scary" world. Although Matthew fought the documentaries at first, he gradually developed them fully in his "Home Sweet Home" and "Learning about Sagebrook" stories. The real world became somewhat less frightening under the protection of the therapist. Matthew then slowly decided to give up the cartoon world totally because of his desire to please and identify with the therapist, as well as his growing awareness of the isolation cartooning caused him. In addition, the real relationships at Sagebrook were beginning to provide pleasures that his fantasy world could not. This process parallels the strides the young child makes within the context of his libidinal attachment to his parents. The initial psychotherapeutic task with many borderline children is to develop a significant libidinal connection within the context of the treatment process. This can be achieved by fostering a connection within the central fantasy life of the child.

The Problem of the Lack of Repression

Clinical Material

After Matthew had successfully controlled his cartoon world, much more direct aggression appeared. Matthew often, in his postcartoon period, broke up the office. He kicked at the furniture and threw toys and crafts around the room. On campus, he seemed to direct his physical attacks toward younger girls, attempting at times to scratch and choke them. Following these open attacks, he would show much self-abuse—throwing himself into the mud, banging his head against the wall, and asking to have his fingers cut off to keep him from scratching.

His theme in therapy was that his "madness" was coming out. The madness came in the form of every-night dreams, dreams that filled the entire night and that he had to relate fully in his sessions. At first, in his dreams, little girls got hurt. They tripped, damaged their knees, and had to go to Mt. Sinai Hospital for an operation. There was, however, a special rock near the hospital; the rock became a rock monster, rolled into the hospital, and bashed and battered little girls until they were all dead.

The little girls, after a period, changed directly into one specific little girl, Matthew's sister, Judy, whom he described as having long, black hair. In his continuous dreams, Matthew tricked his sister into entering a rocket alone. His mother, sensing danger, tried in vain to stop him. The rocket flew into space, crashed into meteorites, and broke apart, and Judy was killed. For long periods, as she rode into space, the wild flight made her scream and yell. There were variations in the dream in which Matthew was able, at times, to trick his mother into entering the rocket to take the fatal trip. In his sessions, he vigorously played out the rocket trip, smashing the rocket against the wall, mimicking the screams, and, at certain points, directly stabbing Judy and his mother after the rocket crashed.

Matthew made many excited side comments as the material flowed. For example, he said "Don't look, it's a very bad game, or "Shut your eyes and don't listen." He could not decide whether it was an adventure or a nightmare, a pleasure or a scare, and he would forcefully fight any interruption of his flow of fantasy for a long period of time. When the therapist attempted to control the outflow of material, Matthew would scream, "You talked, now I don't have time to finish my dream!" "You don't want to hear my dreams"—and this remark would precede a tantrum and acting out in the office. At times, however, there would be an overt plea, "Can you get me into control, Mr. Chethik? If you can control me, I can control the rocket."

During much of this period, Matthew proclaimed that it was very hard to stay at Sagebrook. He felt he could not stand to be there, and he constantly noted he just had to return home. The rocket dreams were often followed by punishment dream episodes. Matthew and friends were chased by mummies (not mommies), and these were biting mummies. They caught the children, stripped them, and bit at parts of their bodies. The children would manage to escape, opening a trap door to the center of the earth. However, as they were going down a long tunnel, lava began to pursue them. As the lava flowed in one direction, the boys turned to run, but the dangerous mummies quickly appeared at the exit.

Discussion

Borderline children often become overwhelmed by their aggressive fantasies. Because of problems in their ego functioning, they are unable to repress (keep unconscious) their primitive rages and sadistic impulses. They feel overwhelmed and experience the anxiety of going crazy ("My 'madness' is coming out," said Matthew). With the borderline child, there is little reflective or observing ego to address one's comments to at these moments. The major purpose of treatment, when this quality of drive material emerges (as it often does with a borderline child), is to *bind* the material and to bring it under some control of secondary processes.

When Matthew gave up a major defense of withdrawal into fantasy (his cartoon world), he had to deal with the split-off, aggressive world he had avoided facing earlier. When he experienced aggression toward his mother and sister (in the rocket fantasies), his ego functioning deteriorated. He regressed markedly into severe acting out of these feelings, and there was a loss of impulse control. His anxiety became overwhelming and, during this period, primary process (primitive) thinking dominated his consciousness. Magically, he feared his thoughts were *actually* hurting his mother and sister, and he wanted the therapist to control his thoughts. The therapist saw, in Matthew, an extensive (though temporary) breakdown of reality testing, wherein he was unable to distinguish between internal thoughts and external consequences. During this period, Matthew experienced a lack of repression, a flooding of primitive thoughts, cognitive disorganization, and concretistic thinking. The therapist used a variety of supportive interventions to help Matthew cope with this disorganization.

Several therapeutic techniques seemed most useful in work with Matthew. At first, the therapist dramatically insisted on talking and commenting on the material, structuring a 10-minute thinking period in each session when the reflective ego processes of the child and the therapist dominated. The therapist pointed to his watch when the therapist (thinking) time would begin. The therapist used Matthew's pleas of "Can you control me?" to show him clearly his fear of the material, his fear of being overwhelmed.

The therapist helped Matthew to clarify internal and external danger, the difference between thought and deed. When Matthew, for example, sought desperately to leave Sagebrook for home, the therapist interpreted his need to reassure himself that his mother and Judy were actually all right. He could then point out to Matthew how often he seemed to make such a big "mix-up"—a really large mistake. He explained that when Matthew came up with strong killing ideas and mind thoughts, he actually became afraid that these ideas would come true in real life. This was a major confusion, a major mistake. How could blowing up Judy in the office hurt her at home? It is important to note that this was done *dramatically* by the therapist. His facial expression indicated incredulity that Matthew could make this confusion; he hit his forehead in disbelief.

The therapist could also acknowledge with Matthew that he was describing many internal angry–killing feelings toward sister and mother. He noted that all children, as they grew, carried not only love feelings for their family but also very great angry, killing feelings as well. When a new younger sister comes into the family, usually boys hate them. The purpose of these generalizations was to provide Matthew with some understandable source for the frightening fantasies and affects he was experiencing (to distinguish them from his term "madness"). They also served to show Matthew that his affect could be a form of accepted and understood communication.

In this period of treatment, the therapist could see the effect of Matthew's weak ego functioning in relation to the aggressive drive. The therapist used a variety of *supportive interventions* to "shore up" Matthew's faulty ego.

Functioning as an "Auxiliary Ego"

Matthew, at first, could not control the outpouring of his aggressive impulses expressed toward sister and mother. The therapist, as an auxiliary ego, insisted on a "10-minute thinking time" in each session, which had the effect of limiting the onslaught of the overwhelming material and created for the ego an opportunity to observe and understand that material. One could say the therapist "threw" his ego into the breach to dam up the flow of instinctual material.

Rebuilding Ego Functions

In this period, Matthew suffered a temporary breakdown of the ego function of *reality testing*. The therapist powerfully addressed this problem by bringing into consciousness repeatedly how Matthew acted as though his internal thoughts (killing ideas toward sister/mother) were having a real effect (he ran to the telephone to find out whether they were all right after his sessions). The effect of confronting and discussing these distortions helped to reestablish more effective functioning. Matthew could observe this distortion in his thoughts as the therapist described Matthew's action.

Using "Binding" Interpretations

The therapist interpreted Matthew's rage toward his sister as the expression of jealousy and a form of sibling rivalry. He explained how little boys feel when a baby sister is born and how these rival, killing feelings were reemerging currently, because he was in an institution and his sister was at home. The purpose of this *binding* interpretation (as noted earlier) is not to elicit more material but to give Matthew a human context and history for these disturbing feelings, in essence, to sum them up.

During this period of work, the therapist needed to work actively and dramatically. It was necessary to use dramatic action (e.g., "You really think, Matthew, that flying your rocket into the wall will hurt your sister?" said with clear disbelief) so that the idea conveyed would be very clear. This process is reminiscent of a mother's making a dramatic point to a young toddler who has done something unsafe. For example, she may proclaim with intense gestures that the stove is "HOT, HOT, HOT!" so that the danger is clear. At points of severe regression the interventions need to be clearly emphasized with borderline children.

The Coersive Quality of the Object Tie

Clinical Material

Matthew, like many borderline children, felt unsafe unless he was in the proximity of an object that he endowed with protective qualities. This need markedly limited his ability to be on his own.

Matthew's limited "reality span" troubled him greatly. He was aware of his need to linger around the child care staff, to touch them at times when he spoke to them, and to be in their shadow. The other boys ridiculed him about this, and he felt the ridicule was justified: his habits did make him feel babyish. Matthew also used the therapist as a protective object. He "touched base" as often as 10 times per day by coming to the therapist's waiting room and feeling close and safe on those occasions. Matthew decided to experiment—he would not visit the therapist's building as often as he had been doing, and when he came for his appointment he was determined he was going to enter through the side instead of the inviolate front entrance he always had to use. No longer, he was determined, would he take the same path going to school every day; even though it was longer, he would try walking all the way around campus. For a period, we found Matthew experimenting somewhat inappropriately—he would suddenly walk out of class in order to try being alone.

On another occasion, Matthew brought in some school problems that seemed to have ruined his day. They had been learning about Paris in class, and he had become very frightened. We came to understand that Paris was in France, and Europe was separated from America by a large body of water. This made his big "getting lost" worry very strong. Matthew's new defenses seemed to begin to go to work as he attempted a new solution. He associated all the foreign landmarks of Paris with familiar landmarks within the United States. The Champs-Élysée was similar to a broad street in Detroit, the Arc de Triomphe was similar to the Washington Square Arch in New York. The Eiffel Tower reminded him of electrical transmitters he had seen near his home. The effect of these associations was to attach the foreign to the more familiar, and the separation anxiety seemed to abate. This was a complex system to make the unfamiliar more familiar, and Matthew began to use it often to cope with object loss. It became an increasingly effective system that allowed him more independence. All trips to new places, which had been frightening earlier, now became possible when Matthew made his familiarizing associations.

Over a period of years, Matthew's reality span, his safety perimeter, grew larger and larger. His earlier need to touch the protecting adult directly became much more symbolic. He came to be able to go on pass into the community, to attend public school, and so forth, as long as he knew that when in a crisis he could reach an adult. He kept several phone numbers in his pocket—he could use them if it became necessary. Again, as all staff became aware of the underlying anxiety that Matthew had with object loss, many devised creative mechanisms that would allow him to take more extensive independent steps.

Discussion

The extremely cumbersome system that Matthew devised to handle his social studies problem (Paris) provided a view of the extraordinary amount of energy necessary for this youngster to cope with object loss. It was, nonetheless, a more effective pattern than his earlier method of attaching himself to his protecting object. By continuing to use this process of familiarizing associations, Matthew was presently able to move further away from his need for direct, immediate "refueling" objects.

How did he develop this greater capacity? Some of the supportive treatment techniques seemed to play an important role.

Confrontation and Clarification Leading to Mastery

Although the interventions of confrontation and clarification are the preparatory steps for interpretation with neurotic children, they can often serve a major function in supportive psychotherapy as steps leading to mastery.

Matthew became increasingly concerned about his pride (he did not want to be called "Baby Matthew"), which was interfered with by his marked separation fears (he clung to staff to feel safe). His conflict (his wish to be accepted was inhibited by his fears) was made explicit to his ego on many different occasions. The therapist drew his attention to the multiple situations in which his "getting lost" worry came to the foreground and how it limited his ability to play with the other kids. As these conflicts were depicted, Matthew sought to master his anxiety by taking measured steps away from the protective object in doses that he could tolerate. Thus, in relation to the protective therapist, he decided to visit the waiting room less often, changed the familiar path to the office, and so on. He was delighted at times that he could control the scared feelings and not run to find the therapist. As his separation tolerance grew, he took further steps. No unconscious interpretation (e.g., his fear of annihilation), as one uses with neurotic children, would have been effective or appropriate.

Dealing with Poor Structuralization

Clinical Material

In the last 2 years of his placement, Matthew made many strides. His academic performance improved; he was involved in some clubs and interests in the community, where he contributed, and although social relationships never acquired an intimacy, he had a few contacts with peers outside the institution. Home visits were pleasurable, and there was a growing reintegration with his family. He was very engaged and busy in his therapy sessions, which he came to use in a particular way.

Matthew developed an extensive system, which he described as "charting." He designed many actual charts with the therapist. Charts were built for school progress, club activity, and mood swings. The graph that followed the course of his moods over the week showed a range from the highest category "calmness" to the lowest category "blow-up," and he reacted with pleasure and received full praise when he had managed a steady, placid week. Acknowledged achievement seemed to serve as a stimulating reward.

The need to anticipate potential upsets, as he extended himself further, became singularly important. Matthew developed an early warning system—What did he need to know to be adequately "on guard"? He made long written lists of potential problems. For example, when summer camp began he anticipated that he might get worried about insect bites, poison ivy, spiders, and so forth. He thought that his "getting lost" worry might come back again. These worries were written down and studied before going off to camp. Before travel vacations with parents he prepared for car accident thoughts, noise of the subway, reactions to tall buildings. A heavy amount of homework and a harsh command from cottage staff were also "on guard"-inducing situations and were written on his study lists. He searched for physical factors as well. He knew he became upset with a stiff neck or sprained ankle, and special watchfulness of himself was necessary at those times.

Role play became an important device to augment his ability to cope with a new situation. He played out how he would react when teased by peers he met in his clubs; he preexperienced sitting through a long church service at home, and practiced and repracticed in the sessions how to find his way to all the classes and the locker room in the junior high he had begun to attend.

Discussion

In this last period of work, Matthew and his therapist developed coping skills that allowed Matthew to extend markedly his perimeter of safety. A number of supportive interventions were used that enhanced Matthew's ego functioning.

Developing Signal Anxiety

One of the major developmental lags evident in borderline children is their anxiety intolerance. Matthew either withdrew from the frightening, anxiety-provoking world or he panicked. In this treatment period, he extensively used trial action, anticipation, and role play, which all helped him develop an "early warning system," a form of anxiety signaling. If he could preexperience frightening contingencies, he would "expose" himself to the new, unfamiliar environment. He also found a growing ability to tolerate stress as long as it came in anticipated situations. He began to use his intellectual capacities to cope with anxiety-producing situations.

Building Defenses

In conjunction with his increased ability to anticipate frightening stimuli, Matthew began to develop contingency plans to cope with these possibilities. For example, if he became frightened of some children in his new classroom, he could walk down to the principal's office. These new rules were memorized, and they allowed him to extend his perimeter. This kind of work in coping with the challenges of growing independence had the quality of compulsive-like defensive systems. He was using his increased intellectual capacity to do this preplanning and mapping out. It allowed him to master his environment adequately for the first time, and it was fostered by his work in his psychotherapy.

SUMMARY

In the process of psychotherapy with borderline children, the therapist has two major tasks. He initially must find an effective way of establishing a libidinal (meaningful) connection. With many borderline children, this means finding a method of *joining* the narcissistic fantasy life the youngster is attached to. (As with Matthew's cartoon world, this process is also described in the next chapter.) The effective alliance allowed the therapist to help Matthew move from his narcissistic world toward an investment in reality.

The second major task of the therapist with the borderline child is helping that youngster with fragile ego capacity to deal with reality. The fragile ego capacity means that the therapist will need to deal with eruptions of impulses, breakdowns of ego functions (reality testing), excessive dependency on the therapist, and a general lack of adequate defenses. This chapter has described a variety of supportive interventions in which the primary goal of treatment was to foster and enhance the ego functioning of the borderline child.

It is important to understand the importance of supportive work with a youngster like Matthew, rather than "uncovering" psychotherapy. For although many of these children have "access" to their instinctual life, the reinforcement of an internal exploration and expression will often promote severe regression. To young practitioners, such an exploration may be very seductive, as it usually involves "good material" (e.g., Matthew's rocket dreams). Most borderline children, with fragile ego resources, cannot tolerate dealing with their internal aggressive life.

BIBLIOGRAPHY

Bettleheim, B. (1971). The future of residential treatment. In: M. Mayer & A. Blum (Eds.), *Healing Through Living* (pp. 192–209). Springfield, IL: Charles C. Thomas.

Chethik, M. (1979). The borderline child. In: J. Nosphpitz (Ed.), *Basic Handbook of Child Psychiatry*, Vol. II (pp. 305–321). New York: Basic Books.

Chethik, M., & Fast, I. (1970). A function of fantasy in the borderline child. *American Journal of Orthopsychiatry* 40:756–765.

Freud, S. (1966). *On Narcissism* (Standard Ed., Vol. 14). London: Hogarth Press.

Kernberg, O. (1975). *Borderline Conditions and Pathological Narcissism*. New York: Jason Aronson.

Mahler, M. (1952). On childhood psychosis and schizophrenia, autistic and symbiotic infantile psychosis. *Psychoanalytic Study of the Child* 7:286–305.

Mahler, M. (1968). *On Human Symbiosis and the Vicissitudes of Individuation*. New York: International Universities Press.

Meissner, W. W. (1978). Notes on some conceptual aspects of borderline personality. *International Review of Psycho Analysis* 5:297–312.

Noshpitz, J. (1971). The psychotherapist in residential treatment. In: M. Mayer & A. Blum (Eds.), *Healing Through Living* (pp. 158–175). Springfield, IL: Charles C. Thomas.

Pine, F. (1974). On the concept "borderline" in children: A clinical assay. *Psychoanalytic Study of the Child* 29:341–368.

Settledge, C. (1977). The psychoanalytic understanding of narcissistic and borderline personality disorders. *Journal of the American Psychoanalytic Association* 25:805–834.

Stern, D. (1985). *Interpersonal World of the Infant*. New York: Basic Books.

Stern, D., & Sander, L. (1980). New knowledge about the infant from current research: Implications for psychoanalysis. *Journal of the American Psychoanalytic Association* 28:181–198.

9

~

Treatment of
the Narcissistically
Disturbed Child

The narcissistic disorder, like the borderline syndrome, has its roots in the separation–individuation phase of development, although it is seen as a less severe disturbance (Mahler & Furer, 1968). Many of the problems evident with borderline children emerge in this disturbance. The narcissistically disturbed child shows similar difficulties in object development. He has a poor capacity for intimacy. The mechanisms of "splitting" of objects into good–bad terms, the processes of devaluation or idealization of self and objects, are commonly evident in this disorder. Many of the early problems of pregenital aggression occur in this pathology as well. However, children with narcissistic disturbances do *not* have the severe ego defects in thought processes, reality testing, and judgment that characterize the borderline disturbance (Settledge, 1977; Boren, 1992). Such children generally have good work abilities and can effectively learn intellectually. These ego capacities allow them to use psychotherapy more effectively, and they are often capable of being treated with a variety of uncovering as well as supportive interventions. It is not well understood what has occurred developmentally that would differentiate these two groups of children. Several authors speculate that with the narcissistic disturbance, the problems occur later in the separation–individuation subphases (namely, the rapprochement sub-phase), whereas problems that lead to borderline disturbances occur earlier in the practicing and hatching subphases (Settledge, 1977; Kernberg, 1984). There is also discussion in the literature whether the disorder is the outcome of insufficient gratification of the normal narcissistic needs of infancy and childhood (the prevailing view [Rothstein, 1977]) or due to an overgratification of these needs (Fernando, 1997, 1998). Tom, the case discussed in this chapter, illustrates insufficient gratification stemming from physical illness.

In this chapter the early psychotherapeutic work with Tom illustrates some of the similarities and differences in the treatment between the two syndromes, borderline and narcissistic pathology. The focus is primarily in three areas: (1) similarities and differences in the developmental histories, (2) similarities and differences in the capacity to adapt to the real world and its demands, and (3) similarities and differences in the treatment process of these two syndromes.

TOM: BACKGROUND, HISTORY, AND SYMPTOM PICTURE

Tom's early life had been dominated by pain. He had undergone constant pyloric spasms during the first 18 months of his life, and all medication had seemed ineffective. His chronic pain had been evident—he grimaced, was often doubled up, and cried constantly, particularly in relation to feedings. He had fought feedings and vomited a good deal, suffered diarrhea, and gained little weight during that period.

Nearly all developmental milestones reported had been delayed or were not achieved at all, especially those in the interpersonal realm. Mrs. G, Tom's mother, recalled no early smiling, no sense of unfolding mother–child dialogue within the first year, no stranger anxiety, and poor attachment behavior. Often in pain, Tom held onto his mother tenaciously, clutched her, and dug his fingers into anything he could grasp on her person. Because of the pain he experienced much of the day, he could make little constructive use of toys. During the first 18 months, he played little with them except to throw them or bite into them. Gross motor development had been interfered with. Tom developed his own unique means of propulsion. In pain, he dug his heels into the household carpeting while lying on his back, and he pushed himself backwards with intense momentum throughout the house. On many occasions, he crashed into furniture.

It is important to note how the parents handled this trying youngster during this period. His mother recalled that she had been unable to calm Tom, and she had felt absolutely terrible about her ineffectiveness. Her self-condemnation was felt even more intensely because her husband could be somewhat more effective, although he had typically been busy and absent. Mrs. G seemed to have been a remote and self-absorbed mother, overidentified with her son and unable to handle him without intense anxiety. She could acknowledge many feelings of her past wish to be rid of this impossible child, and particularly she recalled the desperate longing for some peace from her child's constant irritability.

It was apparent to all members of the family that his extreme pain had abated when Tom was about 18 months old. But the parents questioned whether Tom had ever recovered from the trauma. Essentially from that point on, Tom was described as a "stoic" youngster. He was easy to handle and never made demands on anyone in the family. The parents reported that it seemed as though Tom had developed a "shell-like" buffer between himself and the world.

Tom seemed to erect a characteristic posture that varied little; he was pleasant, compliant, often with a slight fixed smile on his face. Tom never developed any friends. He played near his own older brothers, who developed a protective attitude toward him. He never ventured off the family property, which served as a safe surround and perimeter. Occasionally schoolmates visited him, but neither play nor relationships were sustained, and he seemed to be uninterested.

As he grew to school age, Tom enjoyed reading and devoured a good deal of the extensive family library. Tom developed a positive relationship with his father, but primarily in the form of teacher–student. His father spent much time with all of the children, explaining the natural phenomena they experienced in terms of his extensive scientific background. Tom was evidently quite bright, scoring in the superior range in IQ and achievement tests, yet the same attitude of nonengagement was evident in class. He completed none or few class assignments, never spoke or volunteered in class, and clearly drifted off mentally somewhere during the school day. At times he would also wander back home from recess without comment or explanation to the teacher. He did not arouse anger in the teaching staff; rather, he stimulated rescue fantasies, for although he seemed lost, he was thought to be shy and appealing, and teachers longed to make contact with him.

Mr. and Mrs. G sought treatment for Tom because they had begun to realize that he would not "grow out" of his isolation, and he was falling behind in school because of his chronic lack of investment. In the therapist's early work with Tom, he proved somewhat of a diagnostic dilemma. He did not evidence the generalized ego weakness and the difficulties in thought process that many borderline youngsters manifest, but he seemed to articulate clearly the object relation dynamics generally associated with the borderline syndrome.

Discussion

Tom, like Matthew, had evidenced major problems in infancy. His early feeding pattern was filled with enormous difficulties, and there was evidence of striking problems in the process of attachment to early objects. Thus, he, like Matthew, had experienced the real world as a painful and unsafe place. Both youngsters had utilized severe forms of withdrawal to handle this frightening reality. Whereas Matthew (Chapter 8) had built an extensive cartoon world, Tom had withdrawn into a compliant, buffer-like shell. Tom had "split off" safe and limited areas and had thus avoided the dangerous world outside; the safe perimeter was represented by the boundaries of his home. He had gone through the motions of attending school and associating with peers but had returned quickly to his home and avoided the "hostile" world.

In comparing the early histories of these two youngsters, it is clear that Tom illustrated a quality of ego functioning to handle the perceived aggressive assault from reality that was not evidenced with Matthew. Matthew was generally overwhelmed by stimuli, and his attempts to negotiate his day were very inadequate. He panicked, deteriorated into tantrums, and desperately clung to safe objects.

Tom's ego, in contrast, had appeared able to erect a powerful defensive system at an early age. There had been a massive effort directed at "coping" when, at 18 months, he had withdrawn from the painful world. Tom had erected an extensive character defense to ward off "pain" from objects and the world. He had not been overwhelmed by anxiety; throughout his childhood he had been able to use signal anxiety and to master his internal aggressive impulses. The problem of developing trust and seeing the world as a "good enough" place had remained central for Tom. He had developed a schizoid-like character defense* that had protected him, but this defensive posture had also produced many problems in development. It cut him off from objects and had severely limited his experiences.

TREATMENT

Clinical Material: The Early Work

Tom was a little over 11 years of age when he began psychotherapy. The initial treatment period was dominated by Tom's wooden compliance. He was listless, with little energy, and used a minimum number of words. He made a thin attempt to be serious and appear involved in the ritual of treatment. He volunteered little; in fact, he would go to inordinate lengths to use the specific words and ideas in his answer that the therapist had used in his question. For example, if the therapist noted that Tom had had some problems in school and did not hand in any assignments, he agreed he had school problems, and they were because he could not hand in his assignments or papers. The therapist's words seemed to be safe for him to use. As the hour wore on, the veneer of interchange quickly abated. Tom drifted away, mouthing silent words. With some embarrassment, he would occasionally verbalize them: "Sza, szu Dupres," but he had no associations. Or he would become involved in slowly moving his leg. Again, with some hesitancy, he would describe a complex set of levers that he imagined were controlling and setting his leg in motion. Or he would quickly move his eyes and follow his thumb. He explained that he was not sure whether his thumb moved when he was not watching it, and therefore looked quickly to catch the movements. At first the therapist was concerned about the mechanisms of body deanimation (loss of human features) and fragmentation that Tom was experiencing. However, all of these body preoccupations seemed to be an attempt to organize, order, and explain how his body was integrated. The therapist felt that Tom listened closely when he noted how much Tom was trying to put his body together. When he was very young, he experienced intense and exploding pain (the therapist ex-

---

*"Schizoid-like character defense" is used descriptively. Many narcissistically disturbed children cut themselves off or withdraw into an extensive fantasy world, which serves as an imagined island of protection. This withdrawal separates them from relationships and appears "schizoid-like."

plained the spasms), which must have made him feel he was totally falling apart.

Tom presented a picture of enormous isolation. On the weekend, he could watch 14 hours of TV, and although he had an idea he might go sledding, he dismissed it because his knee hurt. He had a special way of drifting off in school, and he did not know what had actually been said in class. He would fix on the movement of the tip of his pencil and be lost in that fragment of motion. He enjoyed his bedroom and liked to develop plans whereby his sleeping area would be hidden from the view of the doorway; it would be contained as a room within a room within a room. Similarly, he was devising an underground hideaway fort in the woods (though within the property line of his house), which would be virtually inaccessible. He had also been uncomfortable at night as he slept, but he had recently rigged up an opaque shower curtain that surrounded his bed, and he slept more peacefully. Tom, the therapist felt, was seeking to be held, surrounded, nestled, and only then could he rest comfortably. It was as though he longed for the comforting breast without pain. This was indicated by the "womb-like" qualities of his images—the enclosed sleeping area, the room within a room, the enclosed underground hideaway, the shower curtain sealing off his bed. In addition, Tom's history suggested that with the early mother–child bonding interferences resulting from pain, the longing for early comforting might persist.

The Henry stories* the therapist developed together with Tom slowly provided a greater avenue into his internal world. A pleasure world appeared that centered on Sun Valley, an area he had visited for several summers. Henry entered a huge mine shaft and came out, after a long struggle, into a beautiful valley. He lived there in peace, within a small house, and endlessly watched the wildlife, the vegetation, and the light around him. On another occasion he followed the flight of a golden eagle as it soared over the countryside. Later stories included wandering through the woods, touching the deer he had befriended, and walking in the company of two dogs he had known. His stories had no beginning, middle, or end. They were captured still-life scenes that he described in detail. His rebirth fantasy through the long mine shaft led to a pleasure world of pastoral peace and beauty. He seemed to identify with the freedom of the golden eagle, who could avoid and limit his attachment to

---

*Older latency-aged children usually have difficulties becoming directly involved in play, as they feel that play is "babyish." They often develop stories (fantasies) and a story line when the therapist suggests that "imagination" will help to understand worries. This was how the Henry stories came to be born in the work with Tom.

the earth. But there was a strong sense of a total endless pleasure world, his Garden of Eden, where no pain or displeasure ever entered.

The threat to Tom seemed to be the state of being in need, for with the tension of need, an object (caretaking person) was necessary. Internally for Tom, being in a state of need brought back the early feeding, mother–child situation that had brought enormous pain. The Henry stories often led Tom and the therapist to view the Nepal Man. Henry passed this old man, who sat endlessly in a religious trance. Because of his inactivity, he could survive on the juice of one orange every other week. At times when the Nepal Man was going to move his hand to reach out, he would squeeze it in a particular way with the other hand, stop the motion, and create a temporary paralysis. Similarly, Henry passed an old woman who sat trying to thread a needle. Although she was shaking with age, she never stopped and evidenced no frustration or need for help.

When Henry finally turned to people, the objects were typically empty. Henry wandered into an old warehouse that was filled with rusty cans and parts of old tools. He picked them up, one by one, and examined them. Finally he came to a room with a bed in it. When he lifted up the cover, he was confronted by a skeleton in the middle of the bed. "Sir" Henry went back into time to the years of King Arthur's knights. He rode a horse, and facing him on the highway was the figure of the Black Knight. He was still, and Henry attacked with his lance. The knight clattered to the ground, and when Henry lifted the iron mask, there was nothing but blackness inside. On another occasion Henry rode down the Colorado River in his kayak. Vultures circled overhead. He was frightened and moved to a cave for safety. No one lived there, however, and he could only faintly make out the writing of some dead civilization on the stone walls.

Discussion

Tom, like Matthew, recreated aspects of a symbiotic world. At first he had sought to establish an "all-good" world. He had set up a warm surround through his "room within a room" and his underground hideaway. The Sun Valley fantasies, where he was comfortable, were like the protective enveloping objects of early childhood. These appeared to represent times in Tom's early life when he had felt comfort and a sense of peace and tranquility. His fantasy life had the features of the early omnipotent period of primary narcissism. This pastoral world was "all good." Everyone lived in harmony and peace, and therefore there were no demands to stir up aggression.

Tom was primarily attached (cathexis) to this fantasy world, and he went through the motions (like Matthew) in his existence in the outside, real world. Borderline and narcissistically disturbed children, who have problems with objects early in their infancy, develop the need for a safe "cocoon." Matthew constructed his cartoon world where he mastered danger. Tom used his skills to develop his Sun Valley world. It was these internal worlds in which the greatest investment was made, because these controllable worlds provided the greatest pleasure. Minimal investment was made in the outside world. Tom went through school and handled the routine of the day minimally, because reality represented the painful and threatening world. In similar fashion, Matthew had announced "intermission" from his cartoon world when he had to join his peers for activities at Sagebrook.

In the early sessions, Tom also explicated some of the features of the "bad" split-off world. He described the objects, and his people were empty. The skeleton in the rusty warehouse, the empty interior of the Black Knight, the images of the cold cave, vultures, and the writing of the dead civilization depicted Tom's internal representations—the bad objects that inhabited his world. They were cold, dead, and unavailable. These objects represented life in the outside world, and therefore Tom remained primarily attached to his early narcissistic life. The intense negative infantile experiences had fostered this "splitting" into the two diverse worlds. It appeared that when he was an infant, there had been some pleasurable experiences—in being held, for example—and these provided the traces of the "all-good" world. Clearly the "all-bad" experiences had occurred when Tom was fed and he had experienced intense pain. He had been unable to take the important developmental step in childhood of integrating these "good" and "bad" worlds, and the need for "splitting" objects was maintained.

For Tom, to be in a state of need represented a great threat. The Nepal Man lived in a trance but developed a problem when he became hungry (and then needed objects for food). He reached out for food and contact but then stopped himself by "paralyzing" his arm. Tom appeared to relive the early hungry–eating experience in childhood, when he needed to be fed but had used enormous energy to contain himself because of the anticipated pain he would experience.

The Nepal Man was the epitome of the self-contained stoic man, the man who could survive on the juice of one orange every other week. The trembling old woman was a similar self-contained figure who arduously struggled to thread a needle but never turned to others for help. These images were self-representations and ego ideals for Tom. They described precisely the adaptation that Tom had achieved—they created the shell-like buffer between themselves and the real world, even though they did have needs. With the barriers Tom erected between himself and objects, he effectively minimized the pain of the real world. And his daily life clearly reflected the distance he had established between himself and the major aspects of the real world.

Both Tom and Matthew handled their perceived painful worlds by withdrawal into fantasy. However, there were major differences in the quality of their fantasy lives. Many aspects of "secondary process thinking" (the ability to abstract, to use metaphor and symbols) were evident in Tom's thoughts and ideas. Tom had an extremely rich capacity for verbalization and extensive speech, in comparison to the almost nonverbal quality of Matthew's cartoon world. Tom's characters involved extensive use of symbol formation and metaphor rather than the extensive need for direct action that characterized Matthew's play. Creative and synthetic functions were available to Tom, and he could integrate the images of his imagination from his extensive reading and intellectual gifts. Tom had the capacity for sublimation that was not evident with Matthew. It is not unusual that adults with narcissistic disturbances develop successful work and career capacities, whereas borderline adults rarely achieve success in the work area. The difference appears to be in the quality of their respective ego functioning. Matthew's cartoon format had the young child's quality of play where fight and victory (e.g., Popeye and Bluto) provided a sense of magical triumph. This was in contrast to the subtlety of Tom's characterization of the Nepal Man, who represented a complex self-representation in which the issues of food, need, and stoicism were vividly described.

This different level of ego functioning allows the therapist to utilize a greater amount of *uncovering techniques* in the treatment of the child with narcissistic difficulties. During the early period of therapy, Tom slowly experienced greater ambivalence about his extensive isolation. The hours spent in his room, the time away from other people, the solitary perimeter he had developed made him feel "lonely" and "bored" many times. Tom and his therapist began to develop a *therapeutic alliance* in which they shared a similar therapeutic goal. They could commonly attempt to understand the need for Tom's extensive withdrawal from reality and perhaps even alter some aspects of this isolation.

When Tom's "Henry stories" described the idealized scenes of Sun Valley, the therapist began to make both *interpretations* (providing the unconscious meaning of the material) and *reconstructions* (putting these meanings into the context of the past history). He discussed with Tom the comforting world he had had to create and cling to because of the exploding pain he had experienced as a very young child. In contrast to the pain, Tom had constructed a soothing world. And, the therapist added, he continued to create this soothing environment currently by the special surround in his bedroom and the hideaway fort on his property. He acted as though the past painful threat still existed.

When Tom brought out the images of the empty and unavailable objects in his life (the rusty warehouse, the skeleton, the Black Knight, etc.), the therapist again slowly interpreted their meanings. For example, the "little boy" in Tom had come to "learn" (because of the pain in eating) that those who fed him were cold and dreadful and that the outside world was terrifying. Perhaps these past feelings had made him believe currently that all people were similar. Thus he avoided teachers, parents, other adults, and peers and went through the day with a minimum of interaction.

As the creations of the Nepal Man and the trembling old woman appeared in metaphor, the therapist interpreted Tom's enormous fears of reaching out to objects. Both images expressed strong needs for help, but their need to isolate themselves from others persisted. This was exactly how Tom functioned at home and at school. He feared that if he asked for help, he would again experience the intense pain and hurt. This worry came from his feelings as an infant rather than the current reality. These interventions began to produce an important shift, which occurred in the next phase of the psychotherapy.

Clinical Material: The Later Work

The early work with Tom encompassed the first year of treatment. During the next 4 months of work, there was a slow erosion of Tom's complacency and an expanding tension. Tom felt at times like a "caged animal," searching throughout his house for something to do but finding little. He could no longer sit around passively, and his major complaint was his enormous boredom.

Initially, some memories arose. These were thoughts that came naturally. They were of pleasant moments spent with his older brothers. He recalled riding in the back of a truck with them, going into town. He remembered camping with his older brother's friends. He recalled campfires, singing, and the food they ate. He remembered a long walk into town from his home in Sun Valley and how, when he was frightened of the saleswoman in a store, his brother helped him buy the candy he wanted. Clearly, the therapist noted he was now feeling more lonely, and the memories he had were of the few times of loving, close moments with people in his life.

He began to make forays into the city, beyond the perimeter of the land surrounding his home. But he complained that the climate in town was not right. This city was not his kind of place. It was highly polluted, and he longed for Sun Valley. He told of his worries that there were muggers in the city who were out to kidnap him and hold him for ransom, because he came from such a wealthy family. Yet he increasingly drove himself to get into the city each weekend.

Transference elements emerged more clearly in his sessions. Tom elaborated a playful preoccupation that had been growing. There was a major plot going on that pleased him to think about. He was marked for murder. His mother was an important member of the conspiracy, but she would give no indication of being part of this evil group. The therapist was also a member, recently hired, and part of the therapist's purpose was to brainwash him so that he would not be as vigilant as he needed to be. He could be assassinated on any street corner of the city. He imagined himself with a machine gun as he rode through town, blasting away at the attackers. When he walked through the city he carried (in his imagination) a variety of concealed weapons to which he had access to at a moment's notice. These ideas were embellished and elaborated over many weeks. The pleasurable aspect of this affectively distanced scenario was that as he traveled through the city, he was not bored, but in a state of excitement and adventure as he played out these themes.

In new Henry stories, people were now clearly included. Henry found a group of kittens that he took home to care for and nurse. They had been abandoned. But Henry's mother had an intense allergy to cats and would only allow them to be housed in the garage. The result was that they wandered away at night and were lost.

Despite the negative connotations of the indifferent or hating objects, Tom was evidently growing much closer to his therapist. One day, when discussing future plans, instead of talking about his wish to be a

physicist like his father, he slipped and said "psychiatrist like my father." The therapist noted the slip and commented that Tom seemed to
have good fatherly feelings about him. On another occasion, noting that
the therapist had been rather silent for several sessions, Tom said he
knew why the therapist was really being quiet. In a most intense way, he
said the therapist wanted to give him a chance to come out of himself, to
let what was really inside of him emerge. The therapist's quietness,
therefore, was experienced as a loving, interested, and empathic silence.

The newer aspects of the internal Tom were simultaneously filled
with aggression, and there was a growing availability of *real affects* as
he brought forth more internal material. He dreamt of a party where
his mother was preoccupied with the guests downstairs. She came up
to say good night to him, and he noted a bloodstain on her white
blouse. Later he realized that he held a knife. As he described the
dream, Tom clenched his fist and rage permeated his face. Another
dream fragment was of a vampire bat. He commented that although
these bats were seen as ugly and disgusting, among the bats themselves
they were quite acceptable. He then noted that he felt ugly and angry.
In a third dream in this period, he was an observer of a witches' coven
from a balcony. There was much activity within the group as they
scurried back and forth. He realized, as he watched them, that they
were making plans not only to practice evil among themselves but to
affect the world at large. He noted that when he awoke, rather than
being frightened by the group, he was fascinated and liked the idea of
the power they had. He was smart; wouldn't it be terrific if he had the
power to run the world?

Some breakthroughs occurred in Tom's reality functioning. He began to enjoy school and his work there. He felt he now had new energy
for his assignments, and for the first time he volunteered in class. He was
terribly pleased with the fact that when he gave a thoughtful answer, the
teacher smiled and others approved. Several people spoke to him for the
first time, and he was invited to eat lunch at the "popular" table. In addition, he related he did something with his mother he had never done
before. While they were driving, he thought of a funny program he had
seen on television. He wanted terribly to tell someone about it. He related the TV incidents to his mother, and she laughed. As Tom and the
therapist discussed this interchange, it became clear that this was the
first time he could remember bringing something of himself to his
mother. He invariably only answered questions people asked him and
never brought aspects of himself into any encounter. In addition, it was
hard for Tom to believe that he could really make someone laugh—that
he could have a real impact on the real world, mother, teacher, and students in his class.

Discussion

In this phase of psychotherapy, Tom (like Matthew) emerged from his isolated world as it became more ego-alien. Earlier it had protected him, but now he felt like a "caged animal." Therefore, he made forays into the "polluted" city and in doing so began to deal with some aspects of the dreaded aggression he had "split off" and avoided.

What provided the impetus for change and the initial moves out of his isolated world? A major aspect was the effect of the growing positive transference and libidinal (loving) relationship to the therapist. Evidence for this emerged in his slip (wish) to be a "psychiatrist," his comments on understanding the therapist's relative silence at times, the increased sharing of his internal life, and his growing investment in the treatment. The pleasurable relationship with the therapist restimulated the *need* for relationships and underscored his intense loneliness. Thus, the good attachment memories of contact, closeness, and warmth with his brothers emerged in his associations. We can also speculate that his transference capacity to engage with the therapist had an earlier basis—his positive ties to his father. The effect of this experience in treatment was to make him increasingly dissatisfied with the impoverished, isolative world he had created. Thus he became a restless "caged animal" at home, seeking more contact and relationships. But as he attempted to give up his enclosed world, he reexperienced the earlier dreads and anxieties that he had defended against. What would happen when he needed people and sought contact?

What led to the development of the positive transference? Again, it is helpful to use Freud's concept of "repetition compulsion." In the process of psychotherapy, the patient will experience past events that were centrally conflictual and repressed (cut off from conscious awareness). The material in the later work indicates that Tom earlier sought and valued positive and loving attachments, and he recreated this search in treatment. The therapist was then in a position to point out his intense current conflict (a repetition of the past). For example, when Tom brought forth the vignettes about his brothers, the therapist commented that he seemed to enjoy being with other people then, and that this contact gave him a lot of pleasure. Now, however, he seemed to live in a way that really cut off people. Highlighting the conflict contributed to the pressure Tom felt to alter his current separation from the world.

As Tom grew increasingly dissatisfied with his schizoid-like withdrawal, the "unintegrated" all-bad aggressive world reemerged. The city he initially sought to enter was polluted and populated with muggers, kidnappers, and murderers. His mother was the personification of all evil, and even the therapist could become an "all-bad" object joining the conspiracy. The attacking world of early childhood that provided the intense pain reappeared. As the threatening world emerged, Tom at first warded off his internal fears and counter-rage by making a game of his forays into the city. He described *playing* that he carried a machine gun and other weapons to kill the assassins.

As Tom brought on this aggressive world, the therapist had opportunities to make a number of interventions—interpretations of defense and content and reconstructions that were slowly helpful to Tom. The therapist did a significant amount of interpretation linking Tom's vision of the current hostile world (e.g., the polluted, attacking city) to the world he had experienced as a little boy when he felt attacked by the continuous "outside" pain. As he felt he was attaching the past to his current perception of the city, he became less frightened of leaving the perimeter of his home. The therapist also interpreted the meanings of the "plots" against Tom conceived by his mother and others. The therapist linked the current distrust of his mother and her murderous intent to the feelings of a little boy. Tom had constructed, with the pain he had experienced, that he was being poisoned by an evil witch at every feeding. The therapist also touched on the counter-rage any little boy would feel. Tom was destroying all the assassins with his machine guns. When a child felt he was being poisoned, he would not only be frightened, he would also want to kill everyone in sight, and especially the evil witch-mother who he imagined was continuously giving him the poisonous feedings.

One of the major problems facing children with borderline or narcissistic disturbances is the lifelong difficulty they have in integrating the rawness of their pregenital aggression, both emerging from the self and projected onto the outside world (Kernberg, 1984). As Tom became more comfortable with the "playful" game-like murderous feelings he could attribute to himself in the city family, he allowed more real affect to emerge. He experienced the rage toward his mother in the party dream, he felt intensely like the ugly and angry bat, and he vigorously identified with the witches who wanted to rule the world for their evil purposes. The therapist continued to describe the intense feelings of a "poisoned" (perceived by Tom) little boy. The little boy would want to seek revenge against his mother and the whole world. He would seek to bloody (blouse) the clean, deserting mother. In his angry imagination, he would want to become an ugly vampire bat (oral destructive rage) and repay the object world for his early sufferings. Could the witch's coven be his inside idea of the plans the mother-witches were hatching to torture him with every feeding? Tom listened intently to these constructions of his emotional early life.

As noted earlier, as Tom's aggressive fantasies emerged and were made less pernicious through treatment, the real world became less frightening. School, peers, and home became less formidable, and he invested increasingly in his relationships and learning. In subsequent periods of work in the psychotherapy, Tom's intense rage affects broke through, often directed against both the therapist and himself. And as these affects were understood, Tom's investments in reality were further enhanced. In later years, Tom's isolation was significantly altered, but it was the therapist's assessment that his capacity for intimacy remained somewhat limited. For example, he related to peers around interests, rather than to them as people.

SUMMARY

From the two cases described (Chapters 8 and 9), it is clear that there exists a range of severe pathology in childhood. The two children evidenced some similar features in object relations difficulties and in the early separation–individuation phases of development. However, there was a wide difference in ego capacity and achievement in these children. Such differences substantially alter treatability and prognosis. Children like Tom, who exhibit good ego functioning, have the capacity for a significant degree of insight-oriented psychotherapy. Those like Matthew can be helped to master poor adaptation primarily through supportive and ego-building techniques.

In reviewing the treatment process with Tom, we can see many similarities to the uncovering process with neurotic children. The primary intervention was through interpretation and reconstruction. The major difference in work with narcissistically disturbed children is not the modality of treatment itself but the specific content that the therapist needs to understand. He or she must become familiar with the early developmental process of infancy and toddlerhood and the nature of the early interactions with primary objects. These aspects of the early history will arise in the symbolic material of such children (e.g., Sun Valley, Henry stories). In addition, the therapist needs particularly to understand the role of aggression and the adaptation, through the mechanisms of "splitting" and the construction of the all-good/all-bad worlds these children make.

BIBLIOGRAPHY

Abend, S., Porder, M., & Willich, M. (1983). *Borderline Patients. Psychoanalytic Perspectives.* New York: International Universities Press.

Beren, P. (1992). Narcissistic disorders in children. *Psychoanalytic Study of the Child.* 47:265–278.

Fast, I. (1970). The function of action in the early development of identity. *International Journal of Psycho-Analysis* 51:471–478.

Fast, I., & Chethik, M. (1972). Aspects of depersonalization experience in children. *International Journal of Psycho-Analysis* 53:479–485.

Fernando, J. (1997). The exceptions: Structural and dynamic aspects. *Psychoanalytic Study of the Child.* 52:17–28.

Fernando, J. (1998). The etiology of narcissistic personality disorder. *Psychoanalytic Study of the Child.* 53:141–158.

Kernberg, P. (1984). The psychological assessment of children with borderline personality organization. Presented to the American Psychoanalytic Association, New York.

Mahier, M., Pine, F., & Berman, A. (1975). *The Psychological Birth of the Infant.* New York: Basic Books.

Meissner, W. W. (1984). *The Borderline Spectrum.* New York, London: Jason Aronson.

Pine, F. (1985). *Developmental Theory and Clinical Process.* New Haven, CT: Yale University Press.

Rothstein, A. (1977). The ego attitude of entitlement. *International Review of Psychoanalysis.* 4:409–417.

Settledge, C. (1977). The psychoanalytic understanding of narcissistic and borderline personality disorders. *Journal of the American Psychoanalytic Association* 25:805–834.

10

~

Focal Psychotherapy

Thus far the topics in this part of the book (Part III) have focused on children with long-standing developmental problems. Neurosis, character pathology, narcissistic, and borderline disturbances have had their roots in the preoedipal or oedipal phases of development. The purpose of the treatment of these children has been to produce "structural change"—change within the structure of the personality affecting the drives, ego, or superego components. For example, in the discussion of the treatment goals of Fred (obsessional youngster, Chapter 6) it was discovered that his symptoms had primarily been caused by severe superego reactions to his "unacceptable" aggressive impulses. The purpose of the treatment was to produce structural change, to make the internal impulses more flexible to Fred by modifying the long-standing, harsh superego reactions Fred had developed. To achieve this structural change goal, the uncovering that was required necessitated several years of intensive psychotherapy. Similarly, in the case of Matthew, a borderline youngster (Chapter 8), the goal of the psychotherapy was to develop the quality of ego functioning (structural change) that could allow this child to function in the real world. Components of the ego (e.g., signal anxiety, defenses) had to be built through the therapeutic process. Again, this required a period of lengthy psychotherapy. Thus, when we normally think of producing structural change through treatment (altering long-standing patterns of psychopathology), it is almost implicit that the treatment will be both intensive (more than one time per week) and of long duration (usually several years).

There are, however, many situations that children experience that place a strain on their development but do not require extensive psychotherapeutic intervention or major internal changes within the child. These experiences are typically stimulated by focal stress events in the child's life or family life, and they have the potential of derailing the developmental process or have already produced some recent changes in the child's functioning. These are often classified as "reactive disturbances," disturbances in reaction to stress events. The following is a possible list of such events in a child's life, but certainly not an exhaustive one:

1. Death in the family (parent, sibling, relative)
2. Divorce within the family
3. Surgery in the child or other hospitalization
4. Major physical or emotional illness of a family member
5. Major illness of the child
6. Suicide of a family member
7. "Life crisis" of a parent (job, affair, etc.)
8. Birth of a sibling
9. Extensive separations from caregivers
10. Family dislocations

For some children who are well integrated, these events will cause only transitional stress that will be mastered after a period of time. For these youngsters, no professional intervention will be needed. Others will show marked and persistent changes stemming from the crisis. Many children are affected indirectly, less by the event itself (e.g., death of a sibling) and more by the parental reaction. Often there is an alteration of the parent's ability to function as a parent. For example, a depressed mother dealing with the death of a child in the family may have little capacity to deal with the other growing siblings. The parental change may constitute the primary developmental interference for the child.

When it appears that the child's reactions to these events or changes in the parents go beyond a transitory period, an evaluation is indicated, and "focal psychotherapy" may be the appropriate recommendation. This intervention can be directed at the child, parent(s), or both. Typically, these treatment experiences are shorter than those involving children who require structural change, and treatment may last from several months to less than 1 year. The purpose of this chapter is to illustrate this intervention and to discuss generally some of the differences in the process of this work.

THE PREPARATORY PROCESS

All of the aforementioned stress events have been extensively written about in the clinical professional literature. These reports are both general (e.g., typical reactions to divorce, death, illness) and case reports (specific courses of treatment of these children). It is usually very helpful to become familiar with the clinical literature* as one proceeds with the evaluation and treatment of a possible reactive disturbance. In the evaluation process, this can help the therapist distinguish between a transitional reaction (normal) and a pathological one. It can orient the therapist to the specific components of an event that are generally troublesome for youngsters (e.g., loyalty conflicts, reconciliation wishes in divorce). The literature also provides information on how these events will affect the child at *specific developmental stages*. Different developmental stages will alter the child's experience. For example, the extended absence of the caregiving mother because of illness will affect the 2-year-old male toddler differently than the 6-year-old "oedipal" boy. The 2-year-old will primarily struggle with issues of loss and survival, whereas the 6-year-old will be more concerned with affects of guilt about his impulses (sexual, primarily) that "drove" (his perception) his mother away. The 6-year-old will be better able to use other objects (e.g., father) to deal with loss than the 2-year-old who is still in the throes of the dyadic dependency.

In the course of this chapter, two cases are presented, the first focusing on a child who was reacting to divorce and the second on a child who was reacting to the death of a parent. The material illustrates the evaluative process and the course of treatment.

---

*A particularly helpful clinical *index* that surveys the literature was compiled by Berlin (1976). It carries the most relevant readings until 1976.

CASE 1: IMPACT OF DIVORCE

Richard was a blond 6½-year-old boy who had become increasingly depressed and lethargic following the marital separation that had occurred 1 year earlier. The parents described a youngster who was developing well until the family crisis had occurred. For example, Richard had done well in kindergarten and was considered very bright. He now appeared "unmotivated" in first grade and worked below his ability. Although he had many friends in school and in the neighborhood, his wish to play with others had dropped off markedly. He had been an affectionate and cooperative youngster with both parents earlier. He now rarely interacted enthusiastically with either parent, and he had become withholding regarding chores and tasks around both the mother's house and the father's apartment. The changes were striking and appeared related to the marital disruption. In the evaluation sessions with Richard, he was somewhat sad, but primarily sullen and uncooperative. There was clearly a suggestion of intense anger, which he was unable to express directly, verbally, or in play.

Diagnostic Considerations (The Preparation Process)

As noted previously, it is initially helpful for the therapist to become familiar with the available current literature regarding the "interfering" event. There is a considerable body of articles and books on the impact of separation and divorce on children within a psychodynamic framework, including authors such as Wallerstein and Kelly (1980) as well as work by Kalter (1977), McDermott (1970), and Dahl (1993). Generally, divorce is considered a developmental interference that will always create significant internal stress within a child. The child will need to deal with four major affects stimulated by the marital disruption: (1) anger/rage, (2) loss/grief, (3) guilt/self-blame, and (4) fears.

Children are typically *enraged* internally because they feel cheated by the disruption in the family life and their sense of security. The rage may become evident and acted out (for example, expressed by defiance or direct antisocial trends). The anger may feel very threatening, as the child may fear further loss; it may then be defended against intensely (evidence of this may emerge in symptoms such as phobias). One child had to avoid watching TV, because he might see direct aggression expressed, and he would be filled with intense anxiety. The aggressive *wishes* were repressed, and the expression of them (even on TV characters) became a source of fear.

According to the literature, there is usually a substantial *real loss* the child experiences. The quality of the parental relationship with the father (typically the noncustodial parent) changes, and there is also a major loss in the sense of family (Lohr, Press, Chethik, & Solyom, 1981). Direct depression or depressive equivalents emerge within the child and need to be internally handled.

Guilt is a very common affect children experience in the throes of separation and divorce, and usually it has several sources. Most young children have the egocentric fantasy that they were the central reason for the divorce. This kind of self-blame often causes loss of self-esteem (a sense of badness) and a need for punishment. *Loyalty conflicts* very often further the feelings of guilt. It is not unusual for there to be a good deal of rancor between the parents, and many children feel torn between them. Children often feel pressure to agree to disparaging ideas that one spouse expresses toward the other, while at the same time they internally try to maintain a loving connection to the disparaged partner. This struggle causes a sense of disloyalty and guilt.

Many *fears* abound for children during marital separation and divorce. Although they may fear abandonment by the separated father, they are often concerned that the mother will take a similar abandonment course. Thus, we often see clinging behavior and separation anxiety symptoms. The fears of survival are prominent, expressed in concern about money or preoccupations regarding food.

With the preliminary material regarding Richard, what kinds of hypotheses can we generate regarding his internal struggles, which have altered his behavior over the course of the year? Richard is "unmotivated" in school, less interactive with peers, distant from both parents, and withholding regarding responsibilities. Several possible conflicts suggest themselves. Richard does appear to be struggling with his anger stemming from the divorce experience. His withholding patterns in school and at home can be a form of passive aggression, and this is partly confirmed by the sullen, uncooperative stance Richard assumes in the evaluation sessions. Richard would also be struggling with depressed affects that "depleted" his energy to work and interact.

As noted earlier, in this initial assessment process it is helpful for the therapist to refine further his or her understanding about the impact of the event, specifically in the context of the child's developmental struggles. Richard was still in the phallic–oedipal phase of development when the marital separation occurred, and there is further literature that describes the problems of divorce on the "oedipal" child (Neubauer, 1960). The normal oedipal male child naturally competes with his father, and his mother becomes a sexual object. How would a separation and divorce affect a child during this phase? According to the literature, the major developmental problem is that the divorce (typically, the father leaving home) often "confirms" for the oedipal boy that he is indeed the "victor" in this triangular struggle within the nuclear family. Often this victory produces intense anxieties when these frightening wishes appear to have come true. The preliminary material with Richard raised several hypotheses involving his oedipal struggles. Richard appeared to withdraw from his mother, and the close, affectionate relationship disappeared. Did this withdrawal indicate that Richard's "sexualized" feelings indeed became very frightening to him, and he therefore sought to distance himself from his mother? Similarly, we found that Richard's interaction with his father lost its spontaneity since the separation. Did this change indicate that Richard became fearful of the normal competitive feelings a youngster would express with his father? Did the problems with his competitive wishes also inhibit the intellectual progress in school, where competitive feelings are heightened?

The decision was to take Richard into focal psychotherapy to attempt to deal with the impact of divorce, which was clearly impeding his ongoing development. Richard was seen one time per week for a period of 6 months. His mother was seen biweekly, and his father was seen on a sporadic basis (approximately one time per month).

Course of Treatment

In the opening treatment sessions, Richard elaborated intense competitive play. Two army sides emerged, reinforced by tanks, cars, and armored vehicles. Strategy then developed: fake decoy attacks, elaborate spy schemes, smoke screens, and air reconnaissance. Richard also had an array of special weapons that his opponent was without. He had a huge snake that took the entire opposing army to subdue, and it needed the total strength of all the troops to remove the enormous sac from its head; Richard also had a jet streamer, a special plane equipped with flamethrowers that no enemy barricades could stop. And, most powerful of all, he had black monsters available to him who had "poison prickers" that penetrated and stopped enemy soldiers and thereby killed them.

This play gave Richard and his therapist the opportunity to explore a number of themes. The therapist noted how much Richard wished he himself would have a superspecial pricker. When he thought of the super prickers that grown-ups and daddies had, he seemed scared, as this meant that grown-ups had super powers. Richard laughed and noted that only orange juice came out of his pricker. He brought in chemicals from his chemistry set and made many mixtures during his sessions. When the therapist spoke of his wish to have special chemicals in his pricker like daddies, Richard confided that he loved to wet his bed—it was very warm. Whisker, his cat, always slept with him, and that was how Whisker had baby kittens. The therapist could empathize gently, over a period of time, with Richard's wish to be as full-grown as a daddy and do all the things that a daddy did. It was hard for him to still be a small boy, and it made him sad, angry, and scared. Sometimes he had to make believe that he had all the power and that he was the boss.

In this initial work, Richard's intense anxiety over underlying powerful feelings of competition with his father emerged. Richard's envy and fear of his father's power and abilities, represented by his focus on "prickers," was interpreted, as were the accompanying sad feelings of being so little as compared with his father. Clearly, therapeutic work of this sort is common with children irrespective of whether their parents divorce. However, the interruption of an ongoing, emotionally central relationship with his father intensified the conflict and made the fantasies less amenable to new and qualitatively different realistic experiences with father. Without father there to "test out," as it were, the veracity of these fantasies, they retained all of their original force.

Richard then began a long series of stories, which he called "Dungey House." In his stories there was fighting between a mother and a father. A baby listened to the ruckus while he was still in his mommy's stomach. The father did not want the baby, but the mother did. This was the reason they fought. The baby crawled out, smacked the father with his fist, and ran away with the mother to his special "Dungey house." The house was old, broken-down, and cheap. There he tenderly planted a full garden to take care of all their food. He cut wood for the fireplace, and mother and father got a "divorcement." The Dungey stories and adventures continued but often did not have the happiest ending. For example, the police came because the baby was declared a runaway. They put a chain around the baby's neck and took him away, even though the mother fought desperately to save him.

The Dungey stories brought forth one of Richard's hidden conceptions of the marital disruption. He had felt that his destructive behavior and his jealous wishes were responsible for his parents' "divorcement." His beginning phallic–oedipal urges together with an egocentric cognitive view of the world, both in ascendance at the time of the separation, resulted in this self-blame and ensuing guilt. He and his therapist, in the context of the Dungey stories, began to clarify some of the realities of the history of the difficult marriage and parental fighting. The stories understandably ushered in rich oedipal material—his tender and caring feelings toward his mother emerged not only in the stories but in reality as well. Richard also confided that he often sneaked into his mother's bedroom when she was gone and picked the lock of her jewelry box. Then he could see her wedding ring and all the gold that was there.

Slowly, stories that had a different and more empathic view of grown adult men began to emerge in a new series, called the "Old Man Fogey" stories. The Timberlee Hillbillies, a group of young toughs, attacked Old Man Fogey's house. They chopped down dead trees, which crashed against the roof. They threw wood into his chimney, which shocked him and ruined his fire and made his life generally miserable. Yet these were only in the order of pranks. When Old Man Fogey was actually trapped by a fire in the house because of faulty wiring, the Hillbillies climbed on top of each other to reach an open second-story window and rescue the old man. They then cooked a huge pot of soup to warm up the survivor and shared the food together. Richard also introduced a wise old owl in his puppet play, who soothed the impulsiveness of an irrepressible monkey who constantly stole jewelry and who also soothed the viciousness of a primitive father-tiger puppet, who was out to tear the monkey apart. The wise old owl effected continuous compromises, showing the little monkey how he could work and acquire many treasures and teaching the tiger to have some pleasure from the playfulness of the immature puppet.

Other activities became part of each session. There were many highly pleasurable, new-formed, and highly skilled competitive games. Complex forms of tic-tac-toe were introduced by Richard that became furious battles. Moreover, both therapist and child participated in hangman, a special word-guessing game. Richard saved up the longest possible words he could imagine to stump his therapist—"hamburger," "television," "somewhere." And his therapist countered with even longer word puzzles—"sometimes," "nobody," and "Mickey Mouse." And this intellectual battle in therapy had its reverberations in school, where Richard began to work avidly.

Discussion

At the start of treatment, Richard began to have problems dealing with phallic, oedipal, and early latency-age issues that he seemed to have been handling well prior to the marital disruption. He appeared to stop his development commensurate with the age at which he experienced the interference of the parental divorce and the partial emotional loss of his father.

Richard's case illustrates the derailment of development caused by the divorce experience and an applicable form of focal psychotherapy. Richard's initial terror of his own phallic, competitive drives was sufficient to cause inhibitions in both his assertiveness at school and his tender feelings toward his mother. Instead, there was a regressive withdrawal from his mother and an inability to use his intellect at school.

These presenting complaints and their underlying conflicts were seen as related to affects stimulated by parental divorce. For Richard, the affects and conflicts evoked by the divorce included a *sense of anxiety and self-blame* for having caused so major a life event as his parents divorce, *an underlying feeling of intense guilt* over besting his father in the competition for who would "win" (i.e., live with) his mother, an *anxiety over fantasized retribution* for this forbidden victory, and *sadness* over losing his father when he moved out of the family household. An inhibition of phallic competition, the inhibition of affectionate feelings toward his mother, was invoked to cope with these painful affects. The fact of living in a one-parent household with his mother and seeing his father only once a week potentiated these conflicts and made them more difficult to resolve. The reality of living with his mother without father present fueled his forbidden unconscious oedipal wishes and made having affectionate feelings toward his mother nearly impossible. At the same time, when his father became emotionally less central in Richard's life, Richard's frightening fantasies of the angry, overwhelming, and vengeful oedipal father could not be tested in ongoing interactions with him.

There was a very marked shift and growth in a 6-month treatment period. Although the therapeutic relationship had many traditional aspects (e.g., the therapist interpreted the unreality of frightening, unconscious fantasies and the defenses of expressing safe affects to ward off painful affects), the major aspects of the therapeutic relationship had a special quality. Under the direction of the patient, the therapist became an aggressive competitor: At first he was fearsome and terrifying, but with a growing libidinal context in the therapy, the competition in play became increasingly pleasurable and interesting. The feared, vengeful castrations became modulated by the reality experiences with a newly available object, and Richard became increasingly comfortable with his own aggression. He became generally more cooperative and able to use his aggression in learning.

Similarly, in the course of object and superego integration in the therapy, changes emerged through the new attachment. Grown men, who were at first one-dimensional attackers who took little children away with chains around their necks, slowly became full people. Old Man Fogey could be hurt and needy, and Richard could empathize with his pain. The wise old owl in his play represented a strong man who was kindly and thoughtful as well as powerful. Richard identified with the therapist. He became much less harsh in his own superego prohibitions. The self-representation of the irascible monkey does not have to be torn apart by the primitive, angry, oedipal father or locked in jail, but he can be "forgiven" because he is in the process of growing up. Richard's conscience became more tolerant and realistic about his impulses.

These developmental tasks—the greater comfort with the aggression, the resumption of affection in object development, the modulation of superego prohibitions—are the changes that occur in normal growth only if adequate objects are available. Richard could continue this normal unfolding when he united with a new object who served the integrative function his father could no longer provide, within the focal psychotherapy.

CASE 2: A BEREAVEMENT REACTION

Sandra was evaluated at age 8½, a year and a half after the abrupt death of her mother. Her mother had died in a car accident; a friend of the family had been driving the car and had also been killed in the head-on collision, which was the fault of the driver in the other vehicle involved.

There had been a period of shock and numbness (disbelief) for all the family members, including Sandra's father and brother Jason

(1 year younger than Sandra). Memories of the few months following the death were clouded, but the father felt that both children showed moments of intense sadness, weeping, and loss.

Sandra had done well throughout her life. She had been an exceptional student and had had an array of friends prior to her mother's death. Since the demise of her mother, she continued to be able to maintain her high level of achievement, and her functioning with friends and relatives went very well. The past relationship with her mother was described as "close" and "warm," and there were no particular periods in the past that highlighted evidence of tension or stress in Sandra's development.

About 6 months after the death of the mother, Mr. E (Sandra's father) met a divorced woman who was approximately his age. They married after a 6-month courtship, and the two families joined together. Sandra acquired a stepmother and a stepsister, Margaret, who was the same age as Jason.

The impetus for the referral (about 6 months after the second marriage) came from Sandra herself. She talked about being frightened at night and became quite anxious as bedtime neared. She was unable to describe why she was frightened, except to indicate that she feared "bad dreams." Both parents also felt that although Sandra was polite and well-behaved with her stepmother, she maintained a reserve and aloofness from the new members of the family. The parents were disappointed with the continuing distance that Sandra experienced but would continue to let her become "attached" at her own pace.

In the early evaluation meetings with Sandra, she was appropriately apprehensive but relaxed when the therapist spoke generally about how girls are naturally frightened in this new and strange situation. As she approached discussing the night fears, she became visibly distressed and anxious and was unable to describe her fears or show the therapist anything about them in drawings or writing. She indicated, however, that she wanted to have a private place to share these feelings, and she implied she would be able to tell the therapist about her distress gradually.

The therapist recommended a twice-weekly open-ended therapy, as he did not have a good understanding of Sandra's struggle. He felt she was probably dealing with some acute affects related to the death of her mother and the remarriage and thought he could provide a better perspective when he knew Sandra better. The therapist decided to see her several times weekly rather than once a week, because he anticipated dealing with the acute affects that might arise from the traumatic event. He was concerned, for example, about leaving this youngster for a full week with intense grief reactions and anxiety. The treatment lasted for an 8-month period.

Diagnostic Considerations: The Preparatory Process

From the literature on children and death of a parent, there emerges a general consensus that children do not have the capacity to deal effectively with death. Wolf (1958) has indicated that only at age 10 or 11 can children cognitively comprehend the full meaning of death. Wolfenstein (1966) noted that children, if they comprehend death, are unable to mourn emotionally, to experience the painful and gradual decathexis (letting go) of a beloved parent. She noted that they tend to mourn "at a distance" and manage this episodically. Nagera (1980) added that because of the pressure of development, children need to retain their important objects. They will recreate the objects anew, often in idealized form.

In considering specifically how latency-aged children handle the death of a parent (Sandra was 7 at the time and entering early latency), Shambaugh (1961) and Furman (1964) have both spoken of the tendency for children at this age to erect a massive denial. They describe case reports in which all of the affects the children experience related to the death of a parent were defended against acutely. Most authors note that often some intervention is useful to enable the child to experience the dreaded affects emerging from the event and to invest adequately with present or new objects.

What hypotheses can be generated about Sandra at this point? She appeared to be an extremely well-integrated and highly functioning youngster who had a very effective ego. Why was she experiencing anxiety at the present time, 1½ years after the death of her mother? Were aspects of a denial breaking down? Was she attempting to engage the reality of the death of her mother? Was she dealing with the pain of the loss, guilt about the event, or rage about the abandonment? What were the implications of having a new stepmother? Did her needs for mothering from this new object create conflict, inasmuch as they would mean "leaving" her mother and feeling disloyal?

Course of Treatment

After several weeks of treatment, Sandra began to describe an extensive fantasy she had developed that had begun to frighten her. She had created an "at will" (her words) fantasy, meaning she could develop it and think about it through her willingness to do so.

Shortly after the death of her mother, she had developed the idea that she could rise up from bed to contact her mother. She imagined that her spirit had left her body, rose above the roof, above the clouds, and then she would meet her mother. This meeting was located on a large cloud area and had an ethereal quality. Mother characteristically wore a special beautiful long robe, and she also wore lovely jewels. Mother and daughter visited from a distance, and all was totally quiet. They never touched each other, and there was no need for speaking because they could read each other's mind. There was a "glowing" quality to their surround—Mother "glowed" and the house she lived in in the background "glowed." The details of the fantasy had grown, continuously embellished over the past 1½ years.

Sandra was quite upset as she recounted the fantasy world and its history. She was very anxious and spoke almost inaudibly. Things had begun to change. She told the therapist that she was more frightened recently because she was "visiting" more frequently. What had started out as a fantasy that she induced once or twice a week had now become compelling and was something she had to do almost every night. Now she often felt that she did not want to start the dream, but if she concentrated she could hear her mother call her, and she "rose up." The feeling that she was losing conscious control of this fantasy and its production created the terror that forced her to seek help from her parents (i.e., tell them that she was having very bad dreams).

In reviewing this material early in the treatment, the therapist had a number of thoughts. The original function of the fantasy had been the denial of the mother's death. Through the fantasy, Sandra could "keep" her mother with her. This process of denial, as noted earlier, is common with latency-aged children. Through this process, Sandra maintained the object (idealized as beautiful in her glowing gown and jewelry) and also avoided the affects of sadness, rage, and aloneness.

It was also clear that contained within the fantasy was a limited acknowledgment of the death. The union was with spirits: Ghost-like figures of herself and her mother were present, she rose to meet her mother "above" in a heaven-like surround, and there was a lack of human contact, as there was no touching or mutual sounds.

What was creating the frightening shift in the intensity of contact with the mother? Sandra felt greater pressure to join her mother. In the

fantasy, the mother now called her. How can we explain the loss of voli-
tion in invoking the fantasy and the change to a sense of dreaded obliga-
tion? The beckoning of her mother had the distinct flavor of a *conscience call*, and Sandra's superego seemed to be reacting intensely. Did
she originally feel responsible for her mother's death? Were there wishes
within Sandra to "desert" her mother, and did this impulse create intense internal conflict? Did she have to deny her wish for more gratification from real and living objects? It was clear there was internal conflict
within Sandra, and the fantasy now had a punishing quality. Joining her
mother "up above" carried a death (or suicidal) implication, a severe
form of self-punishment.

The therapist's intervention with Sandra was to note generally that
she had developed this dream, or at-will fantasy, to soothe herself, as
many children may after the death of a mother. She had loved her
mother, needed her, and her dream was a special way of trying to keep
her alive. Right now things had gotten very scary with this dream, and
only *slowly* could she and the therapist come to understand together
what was happening. She needed to continue to tell the therapist about
the dreams and her ideas. Sandra continued to draw pictures of her
dreams and the details of this heaven-like setting in her sessions.

During one of the ongoing visits to her mother ("called" by her
mother), a mental discussion between them occurred. Mother wanted to
know how the new mother was. Sandra reassured her mother that the
stepmother was bad and that she still loved her own mother. The therapist noted, at this point, that she seemed to be having a really big struggle. All girls would need, more and more, some *real* mothering in their
lives, but when she came closer to her stepmother, she felt very disloyal
to her own mother. Sandra was very upset. She described how her stepmother recently had bought her favorite luncheon meat, and Sandra had
wondered a little if it had been poisoned. Perhaps, the therapist noted,
she needed to find reasons to keep her stepmother far away.

A great deal of material then emerged about the stepmother, who
was in reality a very wholesome person. At first Sandra was very angry.
She *hated it* when her stepmother *tried* to be a mother. She felt like a
stepchild, blamed for everything that was wrong, and so forth. Holidays
were different—her stepmother was Jewish and she Christian, so they
had to celebrate both Chanukah and Christmas. She was scared about
even mentioning Christ at home. The therapist wondered, from time to
time, whether she had to *make* the stepmother bad, so she could appease
the memory of her mother. All girls her age needed to have someone
close and real in their lives, but she felt this need took something away
from her dead mother. With this form of repeated interpretation, a shift
began to occur. Sandra occasionally permitted herself to sit on her step-

mother's lap and let her stepmother comb and braid her long hair. She had to agree that, for a stepmother, she was fair and did not always favor Margaret (stepsister) in disputes between the children. She liked the gifts her stepmother gave her, especially a soft, feminine pair of gloves. She began to draw pictures for her new mother.

On many occasions in this period, she experienced enormous guilt. For example, she had a negative memory of her real mother—she had not smiled a lot. Sandra confessed her strong attachment to her kindergarten teacher before her mother's death. She even used to have wishes that the orange juice lady (commercial) on television would be her mother, because this lady had a wonderful smile. I noted how all children had times when they wished for other mothers, especially when their real mom was out of sorts. Memories of these natural wishes made her feel terrible because her mother had died, and these bad feelings about herself were especially strong as she was beginning to care for her stepmother.

One of the major affects that adversely effects the course of bereavement is the reaction to past aggressive thoughts and wishes toward the object, the natural ambivalence that all children experience in development. During the preoedipal years, when the mother is frustrating, there are wishes for an "all-good" mother. The natural oedipal triangle involves rivalry and death wishes toward the parent of the same sex. Latency produces the "family romance," longings for perfect parents to replace the natural parents whose faults become evident. These natural past "aggressions" are a common source of intense guilt if a parent actually dies. Sandra clearly struggled with guilt for her past "transgressions" (the attachments to the kindergarten teacher and the orange juice lady), and this guilt was intensely exacerbated by her need for and attraction to her stepmother. This underlying dynamic interfered with the capacity to detach from her mother. She also found a way to use her at-will dream to punish herself for these past transgressions. A formerly soothing fantasy became dreaded and frightening, driven by an attacking conscience.

After 6 months of treatment the "visits" to Sandra's mother came less frequently, and it appeared that Sandra again created the fantasy when she missed her mother. Her acute anxiety toward nightfall abated. In one drawing of the "above" world, there was a sign on her mother's fantasy cottage. It read "HERE LIVES ISABELLE F" (mother's name). The therapist noted that if they removed one letter, the "V," it would read "HERE LIES ISABELLE F." Sandra became acutely sad and told me that she often cried when she saw a car in the street that was the same model her mother had died in.

In the ensuing weeks, Sandra was silent and withdrawn. When the therapist commented on her anger toward him, she told him that he wanted to take her mother away from her. On a recent "visit" to her mother, her mother had told her not to talk to the therapist, who now looked terrible to her, even like the devil. Sandra related a dream in this period. "Old oak trees housed birds and squirrels. A lumberjack came to destroy the tree. The birds tried to peck at the lumberjack." The therapist noted to Sandra that it felt as if he were the bad lumberman who was cutting down the beautiful tree-dream that she had grown and in which part of her was trying to live. The dreams she had developed were used to keep her from feeling very sad about her mother who was gone.

With her stepmother, Sandra began to visit her mother's actual grave site for the first time. She looked at photographs of her mother and experienced much sadness with the members of her family. In the sessions themselves, she recalled birthdays with her mother and special foods her mother had cooked for the children. There were also poignant memories of coming home from school after her mother's death and calling out for her in an empty house. She had called "Mommie, Mommie, Mommie," and heard only her echoes in the house. Some of these memories evoked intense sadness in both Sandra and the therapist.

As Sandra's relationship with her stepmother improved and there were fewer and fewer recurrences of the at-will dream, Sandra and the therapist set a termination date 1 month in advance. For several sessions in this last period, Sandra expressed great anger at her father. She had visited relatives for Easter and had had a wonderful time. They had invited her back and she longed to go, but her father noted that the family had other summer plans. She was furious. She recalled all the good times she had had with her cousins in great detail. The therapist interpreted that he thought Sandra was telling how angry she was with him about the therapy. She had earlier developed a wonderful visit with her mother, and the treatment process had taken away this wonderful soothing time she had had. Sandra obviously had mixed feelings about giving up her mother-dream and the connections she had developed through fantasy.

Discussion

Prior to the death of her mother, Sandra appeared to be doing very well throughout her development. After the death, she attempted to cope with many aspects of the event by developing her at-will dream of union with her mother. Union fantasies with a deceased parent are not uncommon and can be particularly useful for a circumscribed period as the child attempts to come to terms with the reality of death.

Children temporarily use soothing fantasies to deal with all sorts of events. For example, many children experiencing divorce evoke fantasies of reconciliation by their parents to deal with the immediate crisis of separation. Slowly, most children accept the reality of the divorce, or death, and the reconciliation or reunion wishes recede. Sandra's union wish with her mother, however, was not abating, and she had been brought into treatment because it was indeed intensifying.

The persistence of the fantasy appeared to be fueled by several internal factors. In part, it was driven by Sandra's *intense guilt*. She had felt very guilty about some of her earlier natural ambivalence toward her mother, as well as her attachment wishes toward her stepmother. Any internal wish to separate from the mother (give up or lessen the fantasy) appeared to evoke enormous guilt, and Sandra denied her wish to separate by intensifying the tie. Another factor that fueled the fantasy was her fear of the affects of *sadness* as she experienced loss. To actually acknowledge the grave, the memories, the car model her mother had died in, evoked intense sadness, which was very frightening to Sandra. Keeping mother alive in the dream warded off these affects and the sense of emptiness and aloneness she experienced without her mother (e.g., the memory of calling for her mother in the large empty house).

Earlier it was noted that focal events have the potential for "derailing" the natural developmental process. Richard, 1 year following his parents' divorce, showed inhibitions in school and withdrew from his parents. With Sandra, there were no manifest symptoms or behavior difficulties 1½ years after the death of her mother, except that she experienced a growing subjective anxiety. It is clear that although she functioned well, the death (focal event) had the potential for significant developmental interference that had not, as yet, manifested itself.

What problems could have developed within Sandra if there had not been some intervention? It appeared as though Sandra was in the process of constructing a *harsh and punishing superego* as a reaction to the death. Her guilt regarding her "disloyalty" toward her mother was corrosive, and it was increasingly interfering with her life. Her growing need to join her mother above (evoked by her guilt) had an element of a death wish, which her conscience appeared to be stimulating. It appeared, in the course of treatment, that Sandra's "confessions" of her affection toward other objects (teachers, orange juice lady, stepmother) allowed her to modify her intense disloyalty guilt.

Similarly, what would have been the potential impact on Sandra of the extensive use of denial (of the death of the mother)? The vividness of the fantasy and the growing incursion on her daily life raised questions about potential problems in *reality testing*. Could the need for mother (both gratifying and defensive) have fostered a growing investment in the fantasy world that would have rivaled her commitment to reality? It was also clear that the dream world that was erected could severely interfere with her ability *to invest in her new maternal objects*. She clearly needed to distance herself from any "replacement" object in order to maintain her loyalty to her mother.

Because the mourning process could not be completed in this stage of childhood, Sandra would need to continue to work through her grief at other stages as well. Separation from home, going to college, and marriage might be nodal points in the future, where this youngster and the young adult could again face conflicts involving her early childhood loss. The possibility of the need for further work in the future was shared with Sandra and her parents.

CONCLUSION

How does the process of focal psychotherapy compare with long-term treatment? The treatment experiences described in this chapter were quite similar to the work with neurotic children, except that they were shorter in duration, moved more quickly to the underlying central dynamic issues, had less protracted periods of resistance, and the changes in symptoms or behavior difficulties occurred more quickly.

One general issue in work with children with reactive disorders is that it may be difficult for the therapist to sort out for a long period of time whether this is a case in which the child is reacting to a focal event or indeed has a form of a more extensive psychopathology. Is the child reacting to an acute stress, or is there a more extensive problem? For example, this was a nagging question in the work with Sandra. When the history was explored, the therapist had questions about its thoroughness and accuracy. On one hand, the major history provider (the mother) was absent, and on the other, the therapist wondered about the general need of the family to idealize the memory of the mother as a caretaker. Individuals who die are often recalled in idyllic terms. As the case unfolded, there was material that made the therapist wonder about the possible harshness of the real mother. Was the perception that Sandra recalled of the mother never smiling a real perception or a distorted one filtered through the child's natural ambivalence? Why did she have to "cling" to her mother so tenaciously? Was she defended against her natural ambivalence (the premise the therapist used in the work), or was the ambivalence exacerbated because of a problematic mother–child tie? These are common concerns that child therapists struggle with in work with reactive disturbances.

Focal psychotherapy does not imply altering a basic insight-oriented treatment process. In these cases the processes of confrontation, clarification, and interpretation were absolutely necessary to achieve resolution of problems. Sandra came to understand the frightening, aggressive impulses she had toward her dead mother that had been repressed. Richard experienced aspects of his competition with his (noncustodial) father in the transference that had created inhibitions in his work and phallic development. These issues were fully explored, as in a long-term therapy.

Because children with reactive disorders have a relatively healthy history in development, they often evidence facets in their personality that foster an effective and rapid treatment process. Both Richard and Sandra formed positive working relationships quickly that supported the treatment process. Many such children have had a history of solid object relationships before the developmental interference and therefore have developed a sense of "basic trust" before the problematic events in their lives. These children usually do not have the rigid defensive postures that are in evidence in children with long-standing problems. Although Sandra used the defense of denial in relation to her mother's death, this was not a mechanism she used extensively in her character. The resistances do not have the protracted quality seen in more disturbed children. Therefore, with the assets these youngsters had through their earlier development, they were able to regain an effective developmental course through a shorter treatment experience.

BIBLIOGRAPHY

Berlin, I. N. (1970). Crisis intervention and short-term therapy: An approach in a child psychiatric clinic. *Journal of the American Academy of Child Psychiatry* 9:595–606.

Berlin, I. N. (1976). *Bibliography of Child Psychiatry*. New York: Human Sciences Press.

Dahl, E. K. (1993). The impact of divorce on a preadolescent girl. *Psychoanalytic Study of the Child* 48:193–207.

Furman, R. (1964). Death and the young child. *Psychoanalytic Study of the Child* 19:321–333.

Kalter, N. (1977). Children of divorce in an outpatient psychiatric population. *American Journal of Orthopsychiatry* 47:40–51.

Lohr, R., Press, S., Chethik, M., & Solyom, A. (1981). Impact of divorce on children. The vicissitudes of the reconciliation fantasy. *Journal of Child Psychotherapy* 7:123–136.

McDermott, J. F. (1970). Divorce and its psychological sequelae in children. *Archives of General Psychiatry* 23:421–428.

Nagera, H. (1980). Children's reactions to the death of important objects. In: H. Nagera (Ed.), *The Developmental Approach to Childhood Psychopathology* (pp. 363–404). New York: Jason Aronson.

Neubauer, P. (1960). The one-parent child and his oedipal development. *Psychoanalytic Study of the Child* 15:286–309.

Proskauer, S. (1969). Some technical issues in time-limited psychotherapy with children. *Journal of the American Academy of Child Psychiatry* 8:154–169.

Proskauer, S. (1971). Focused time limited psychotherapy in children. *Journal of the American Academy of Child Psychiatry* 10:619–639.

Shambaugh, B. (1961). A study of loss reactions in a seven-year-old. *Psychoanalytic Study of the Child* 16:510–522.

Wallerstein, J. S., & Kelly, J. B. (1980). *Surviving the Breakup*. New York: Basic Books.

Wolf, A. K. M. (1958). *Helping Your Child Understand Death*. New York: Child Study Association.

Wolfenstein, M. (1966). How is mourning possible? *Psychoanalytic Study of the Child* 21:93–123.

IV

~

The Process
of Treatment:
An Elaboration

Introduction

In the forthcoming two chapters in this book, two cases are presented: the treatment of a 5½-year-old boy and the treatment of a 7-year-old girl, with attendant parent work in each case. These reports are much more extensive than those of cases presented earlier. The purpose of this elaboration is to bring the reader much closer to the intimate process of treatment: to have the reader experience the step-by-step interaction of the therapist and child in the treatment hour, to extensively provide the therapist's thinking at the moment (printed in italics in the text), and to allow for a fuller discussion of the use of play and other techniques as they emerge in the case.

An area touched on earlier in the text is the importance of the developmental framework as we evaluate and treat children. Many of the cases described earlier had arrests and fixations in the early psychosexual phases of development. To assess pathology, to assess progress in the on-going treatment, the practitioner needs to use the backdrop of normal development. It is beyond the scope of this book to provide a general developmental framework (the reader is again referred to Tyson and Tyson, *Psychoanalytic Theories of Development*). Because the two cases presented fall into the oedipal and latency phases of development, I illustrate how a therapist takes the developmental context into account as he or she works.

11

∿

The Case of Andy B

INTRODUCTION: THE OEDIPAL YEARS

The material in this chapter focuses on the evaluation and treatment of a 5½-year-old boy. The diagnostic process is presented initially, followed by the unfolding psychotherapy. The discussion of the psychotherapy includes the early, middle, and ending phases of work with both the child and the parents.

As noted earlier, prior to focusing on an individual child patient, it is imperative that the therapist have a general context, or a backdrop, within which to place this new patient. What can we normally expect of a 5½-year-old youngster? What *developmental considerations* are paramount for boys and girls this age?

We would anticipate that a 5½-year-old is in the midst of his oedipal years. Internally, in this phase of development, the child is at the height of experiencing his infantile sexuality (Freud, 1905). He is preoccupied with his growing body and the genital excitements he is feeling within it. He has recently become aware of the differences of the sexes, and he struggles with a variety of "theories" about how babies are made, how pregnancy and birth occur. Genital pleasures abound, and masturbation is a common phenomenon. Such preoccupations are occurring even if they are not readily observable by parents or other surrounding adults. Many of these affects cause anxiety, thus they can be defended against and remain somewhat hidden. The oedipal child sees the world from a body-centric perspective because, during these early years, the child's bodily needs and sensations are a primary source of his thinking and motivation. His sexual preoccupations serve several functions—they are a source of pleasure, but also a source of learning about the self and relationships with others (Freud, 1908).

For a youngster in this developmental period a significant aspect of his sexuality is naturally directed toward major figures in the environment. The young boy typically seeks out or thinks about his mother as a sexual companion. He is a young, loving suitor, but this is complicated by the factor of his growing awareness of a triangular quality in his major relationships. Father stands in his way and becomes a rival, an individual he perceives as having rights and privileges with his mother that he does not possess. There are also many other features of the oedipal years. The father's rivalry raises intense fears of retribution, which we typically discuss under the concept of "castration anxiety." In addition, the young child is slowly incorporating many prohibitions into his developing conscience, and thereby the aspects of shame and guilt, internally stimulated, are developing. Thus, the oedipal years are a period of natural turmoil in which the child struggles with his rivalry and jealousy, guilt over his intense sexual wishes, and anxiety regarding punishment (Freud, 1924).

As we anticipate evaluating a young girl or boy, how will the child's specific problems fit into this underlying developmental framework? Has he allowed his genital sexuality to emerge, or does he cling to earlier developmental phases? Are his major conflicts developmentally appropriate? If he is struggling with oedipal issues, is he having particular trouble negotiating some aspects of these normative conflicts: Are his anxieties excessive? What supports does he derive from the family? How does father cope with the childhood rivalry of his son, or mother with the "advances" of the young suitor? How much of the turmoil in each case will reflect the transitory conflicts of a typical "infantile neurosis" (Nagera, 1966) within a 5½-year-old boy, or reflect entrenched conflicts that could lead to a long-standing disturbance?

The natural conflicts described here are gradually worked out, abetted by the child's capacity to play out these issues. Children between the ages of 4 and 6 typically have extensive fantasy lives that help them to master these issues. In nursery schools, oedipal play is often observed. A little girl becomes a mother, and she is very involved in all aspects of caring for her little child doll. She changes diapers, feeds and soothes the infant. In her imagination, she is temporarily not a little girl, but a full-blown woman who has a baby of her own, a coping denial. The phallic little boy carries around a huge sword and powerfully subdues hairy giants. In his imagination he temporarily is a powerful man, more powerful than the adult male father—another coping denial. Gradually, during the oedipal years, the play shifts. The little girl becomes the teacher, and the boy a powerful baseball player. They give up the direct rivalry with their parents and become imagined contributors to society, standing with their parents. In the preceding examples the function of play helps these children make important accommodations. At first they can express these intense rivalries in play, then gradually substitute future "adult" pleasures in union with the former rivals.

The Evaluation of Andy B and His Family

The evaluation consisted of three interviews with Mr. and Mrs. B and two meetings with Andy, in which the basic material was gathered. This material included a discussion of the presenting problems, the developmental history of Andy, a discussion of each parent's original family and background, and some review of the new family's development. A follow-up session occurred in which the results of the evaluation were shared with the parents and then with Andy. The B family was an intact unit. The B's were in their mid-30s and had been married for 10 years. Andy was the oldest child, and he had one younger sibling (Mary) who was almost 3 years of age. Both parents were professionals and lived in their own one-family home in a middle-class neighborhood.

Presenting Problems

Mr. and Mrs. B said there were "crises" with Andy every spring, starting when he was a little more than 3 years of age. During that first spring, Andy began going to a play group three times each week. This was his first separation from home and mother. He had a very difficult time, was frightened of going, and began to develop some sleep problems. He had many dreams each night in which he said he "couldn't find mommy." He would wake up, or be fearful of going to sleep. This distressed state disappeared after several months. The parents were aware that this crisis emerged shortly after the birth of Andy's sister and linked this event to the separation problem.

As I enter an evaluation, I am always aware that resistance abounds as parents discuss their child's symptoms and history. They will distort the history, forget meaningful material, repress events in an effort to present themselves in the most favorable light. These are understandable distortions, and I have found it important to systematically "cross check"" the information I am receiving. For example, the parents say that the difficulties with Andy began at age 3. In my history taking, I will fully inquire about infancy and toddlerhood and not accept at face value that the origins of Andy's difficulties began during his third year.

The following spring, the parents noted that Andy (now 4 years old) became directly aggressive with Mary. He was intensely "on her case," criticizing her constantly, getting in her way, and physically pushing her. He began taunting her with "Ugly face," a remark that upset her a great deal, but he claimed it was "only a joke."

During the most current spring (at age 5—the evaluation was done in the fall), Andy's difficult behavior reemerged; it was no longer transitory, and Andy's parents felt he was quite troubled. He had lost his playfulness and good humor. He seemed angry all the time at Mary and his mother. The parents had to be vigilant now, because Andy could hurt Mary. He teased and "name called" throughout the day. Sleep problems returned, and Andy often showed evidence that he didn't like himself. He often said he didn't deserve to live and he should go to "H" (unclear whether this was a reference to heaven or hell). Night terrors came four or five times each week. The parents reported that Andy had said, "Mom, in this family you hate me the worst because of what I do to Mary."

Andy openly discussed hating Mary and said he wanted to live with another family. He wanted to move into his neighbor's house, which had three boys but no girls living there. He also became preoccupied with the subject of death and burial. "What happens to your body and bones?" he wanted to know, but he became very agitated when there was an attempt to discuss some of his questions. At times, in recent weeks before the evaluation, Andy would sit and rock or repeatedly bang his head—a behavior his parents had never seen before. This acute display of distress and regression alarmed the parents and precipitated the referral for treatment.

In accumulating information it is always important to move be-

*yond the general statements of parents and to focus on specifics.
Thus, when the B's say, "He is angry all the time" or "He hurts
Mary," I invariably ask for examples. I ask, "How so? Can you give
me some illustrations?" or "What kind of things does he do?" It is
not unusual for parents to be unduly anxious about a child's "aggression" or, conversely, to dismiss serious manifestations of pathology.
Therefore, their general impressions may be distortions of the relative normality or pathology of the problems presented, and the specifics clarify the issues.*

*Parents also have difficulties discussing how they handle prob-
lematic behaviors and their own reactions to their children. I sensed
that Mrs. B felt fairly comfortable telling me about Andy's interaction with Mary, but that it was harder to discuss her own relationship with him. Therefore, when she said that Andy was angry with
her, I asked specifically what he did. It then emerged that he was defiant, stubborn, and willfully disobedient, and his mother had a tendency to become internally angry and frozen and to avoid a direct
showdown. This was clearly an important presenting problem, but
unlikely to emerge without my specific probing.*

*Thus far in the evaluation, I had a growing picture of this
youngster's pathology, but little sense of his overall strengths. I felt I
needed to know more about his general ego functioning. I spent time
asking questions about self-care (dressing, eating, cleanliness), friendships, and skills.*

Although Andy's behavior seemed to be deteriorating at home,
there were many areas of strength. Andy had a great deal of pride in
his room and possessions. He collected all kinds of trading cards,
sorted his collections avidly, and traded skillfully with friends in the
neighborhood. He was interested in the current fashions that boys
wore to school (gym shoes, baseball caps). In fact, his parents
thought he had good taste in his clothes and his color arrangements.

Andy ate well, had good table manners, used his utensils appropriately, and was willing to try new foods. He was interested in many
different athletics and developed skills in gymnastics and soccer.
There was also little question that Andy would become a good student. Reports from nursery school and kindergarten consistently indicated that Andy learned well and had many friends in school.
There were no problems in kindergarten, in either his social or academic functioning.

Some of my earlier concerns about the extensiveness of Andy's problems were ameliorated as I collected this positive material about his general functioning. Therapists tend to be pathology oriented and often ignore critical material that can provide a more accurate picture of a child's functioning.

Developmental History

The parents married in their mid-20s. The mother was an elementary school teacher, and the father an engineer. They waited 5 years before they decided to have children because the mother wanted to continue teaching and they wanted to build a "nest egg" so the couple could buy a home and make other major purchases. When these goals were achieved, they started a family.

His mother did not work during Andy's early years. She actually began to work half-time when Andy was about 3½ years old because his father was experiencing a temporary period of unemployment. During Andy's early years, his mother described having a feeling that she could never be as close to anyone as she was to him. She loved feeding him, washing him, playing with him, and felt he was always responsive. He ate and slept well and was typically in a good mood. As the mother related this material, the events she described were vivid and her sense of pleasure was clearly conveyed. However, as the mother began to describe the toddler stage, she became anxious and wanted to move quickly to the later birth of Mary. I noted her anxiety and brought her back to the active 2-year-old. She was markedly uncomfortable as she described the events of that period. She worried that Andy would become too much to handle. His father had little difficulty saying "No," but his mother recalled feeling very tense as she tried to establish rules about climbing on the furniture and cleaning up toys. The father was the person who toilet trained Andy without any trouble; the mother felt that she faltered and that Andy would not perform for her.

It was interesting to note that the difficulties in the toddler area were recovered because of the evaluation process. The family story hitherto was that Andy's difficulties began with the birth of Mary. This underscores the need to fully explore the history rather than accepting the preconceived (perhaps well-meaning) version of the parents.

At about the time of Mary's arrival in the family (when Andy was 3½), tensions started for the B's. Mr. B began to have trouble at work with some of his supervisors, and this ultimately led to his dismissal. The new arrival was an extremely difficult child. She, in contrast to Andy, was agitated, angry, and unresponsive and seemed to have a characteristic "scowl" with which she greeted the world. She would often avoid eye contact with her parents and had trouble in all routines, including eating and sleeping. Both parents described vividly the distress they felt and said that it took an enormous effort on their part to make and sustain an affective attachment with Mary. They often said that in those difficult times, they were blessed with a "lemon" in their second child. By age 2, Mary seemed to overcome the troubles of her earlier years, and both parents proudly felt she was doing very well. They noted parenthetically that Andy's problems seemed to develop in this period.

During these oedipal years, according to the parents, Andy had shown no sexual interest or curiosity and they had not observed him masturbating. However, they were currently aware that Andy exchanged "bad words" with the neighborhood children. There was no evidence of any rivalry with his father or special love wishes toward his mother. Actually, in recent years, much of the earlier loving time between mother and child had vanished, and Andy was often upset and angry with his mother. He wanted and accepted comforting at various times, but showed little of the spontaneous affection he had exhibited earlier.

As we explored this material, it was clear that the parents were uneasy about sexual matters, and they acknowledged as much. I could see the tension in both parents as I tried to discuss masturbation, nakedness, and the sexual curiosity we see in children. The mother also related that she was uncomfortable with Andy's "rambunctiousness." She thought she felt more comfortable with the tea sets and dress-up clothing that Mary loved. The noise of Andy's trucks banging into the furniture jolted her. She mused in the interview, "Maybe I don't understand boys."

At this point it was clear to me that the parents contributed to some of Andy's difficulties. Mother showed some discomfort with Andy's rambunctiousness during the anal phase of development, prior to the sibling difficulties. I felt this could be linked to Andy's current defiant and fighting pattern with his mother. It also emerged that there was a lack of oedipal development. Both parents may have contributed to this problem because of the difficulties they had in accepting the normal (and intense) sexuality of childhood.

I also felt during these initial meetings that I was beginning a "process" with the parents. The B's, like many parents, wished to focus only on the child, and not be seen as "patients" themselves. Too often child therapists comply with this implicit wish. As I focused on their internal reactions to Andy and explored the anxiety and discomfort they had experienced during different developmental phases, they began to discover their specific contribution to Andy's difficulties. Thus, I was developing the foundation for a treatment process for the parents as well. As I explore further, will I find some issues in the parents' background and family of origin that affect their ability to parent?

Parents' Background

Father. Mr. B, an only child, grew up in an upper-middle-class family where both parents were college professors. They taught at a university in a small college town, and Mr. B felt there was a sense of stability and order in his life. His parents were scholars—fastidious and well organized—and he believed that he had adopted these traits within himself. He recalled liking his home and friends and always working hard to achieve in school to please his parents and himself.

Both parents died when he was in his early 20s. He felt alone, isolated; he lived away from his hometown and had very little extended family that could provide a sense of roots.

The father seemed quite sad as he discussed his childhood. I wondered whether he had adequately mourned these early losses. As he described his fastidiousness, I wondered how he reacted to his "unruly" son.

Mother. Mrs. B also came from an upper-middle-class family and was the fourth child in a sibship of five children. Her father ruled the family—his authority was absolute, though he never used force. A meaningful look was all that was needed. He was also very achievement oriented for the family: There were major academic and social goals.

Mrs. B thought her mother was wonderful—devoted, energetic, warm. The parents of Mrs. B felt enormous pride that their large family was extremely well behaved. The children never scrapped; they listened to all the rules and were always helpful to each other.

Mother and father expected that. As Mrs. B related this information, she had intense reactions. She said that she had felt, for some time, that she and her children do not, *at all*, live up to these standards of her family of origin. On one hand, she wondered whether she was a failure. On the other, she thought perhaps these standards were unrealistic. I suggested that it might be helpful in the future to explore some of these ideas.

Courtship and Marriage. The B's met in college. The mother felt she was always shy, and the relationship was the first substantial boyfriend–girlfriend relationship for each of them. They both felt content in the marriage. They shared the idea that the family was more important than their careers, and they were concerned that they were failing somehow to provide the quality of family life they desired.

Contacts with Child. In the course of the evaluation, I saw Andy for 2 sessions. He impressed me as a well-developed, robust, well-put-together young man. He was well groomed and well dressed, and although this was a new situation for him, he seemed relatively comfortable and trusting. He told me his parents said that I was a "worry doctor," but he wasn't sure he had any worries. He separated easily and was relatively nonverbal in his play. However, he became intensely involved in the play story that unfolded.

Andy took to the Legos immediately and elaborated the following play for both sessions. A bad guy (a crook) broke into a house and stole jewelry. He was caught by the police and placed in jail, from which he would escape only to steal again. (With my help, Andy built a jail, a house, a helicopter, and police cars to apprehend this criminal.) After each new crime, he was brought before a judge (a scene that we acted out together, under his direction). The judge sat on a high throne and gave harsher and harsher punishments—10 years in jail, 20 years, 50 years, and so on. No matter what was done, the criminal activity continued.

The major affect (a fleeting smile) occurred when I played the role of the judge (under Andy's direction) and acted harshly and angrily and expressed exasperation with the elusive, unrepentant criminal, who escaped once more. At one point during these sessions, I talked about the "stealing feelings" (impulses to take things) that all boys had. Andy told me he stole money and chewing gum from his mother's purse.

In this initial sequence in the evaluation, I "join" the play. I help build the equipment that Andy wants for the police station, and I act out and animate the role of the judge under his direction. My voice is deep with authority; I express frustration and exasperation for the criminal's repeated acts. In this way the therapist becomes a player, acting out roles as children do together. In this doing this, I give notice to Andy that I can speak his special language.

This play engagement is not an easy step for many child therapists. It means some shedding of the adult verbal role; it means some regression in the service of the ego and calls for some creativity in play on the part of the adult. There are often natural inhibitions that therapists feel at first.

Psychodynamic Technical Assessment

The purpose of a comprehensive assessment is to shed light on the problematic areas (some of which may not be evident from the presenting symptoms alone) and to explicate the underlying forces that have created the difficulties. Andy presented several issues:

1. The major manifest difficulty consisted of the open anger and fighting relationships that Andy had developed with his sister and mother. He was angry with them all the time. This was expressed by hitting and verbally attacking his sister, and by verbal assaults and defiance of his mother.

2. There was a growing problem with anxiety. Andy seemed increasingly distressed, evidenced by rocking and loss of pleasure in play. The rocking behavior appeared to be an attempt to self-soothe when he was acutely anxious. His nightmares and sleep problems continued, and he was becoming preoccupied with death.

3. This anxiety state was accompanied by a growing loss of self-esteem. He felt he should be sent to "H" (heaven or hell) and that he was the "worst boy" in the family. He began to bang his head as an expression of his self-hatred.

4. An area that was not initially presented, but emerged in the evaluation, was the lack of phase-appropriate (oedipal) behavior that would be expected at this age. The assessment showed little of the sexual preoccupation and interests of the 5- to 6-year-old and none of the "suitor" behavior toward mother or rivalry with father.

This omission or gap in development should be considered a presenting problem, although not experienced as a concern by the parents.

I. Drive Assessment

There was a good deal of evidence that Andy had reached the phallic level of development. There was a general "boyishness" about his behavior, and he sought out sports and competitive games with boys in his neighborhood. He clearly preferred male activity, shunning play with girls. Although the phallic behavior was evident, I saw little of the oedipal features that would be expected. As noted earlier, although Andy exhibited many masculine features (phallic), there was no "triangulation"—rivalry with his father and sexual interest in his mother.

There were many problems in the development of the aggression drive. Andy was openly angry with Mary and his mother, and this anger seemed to exceed, in quantity, the anger that one would expect in a normative sibling rivalry or a normative mother–son relationship. In quality, the form of the anger had pre-oedipal (anal) features, inasmuch as cruelty, fighting, and control battles (with mother) were prominent. It was also interesting to note that these anal features appeared to shape the nature of Andy's object tie with his mother. He was fighting, defiant, and controlling, and this behavior had few of the elements of tenderness, caring, and "romance" that one usually notes with an oedipal youngster. Another feature of Andy's aggressive drive was that it was turned inward. He directed rage against himself, evident in his self-castigation, nightmares, fears, and head banging.

Although I saw some problems in drive development (both sexual and aggressive), they had to be seen in the larger context of adequate development. It was significant that Andy's problems with aggression were confined to his home and self. Andy was not generally aggressive in school or in the community. Although he showed problems in his object tie with his mother, many of the standards and values intrinsic to their relationship had been internalized, because he functioned very well with other adults and peers. Some anal fixation points and regression from oedipal phase development were noted, but at the same time much of Andy's general drive development was well developed.

II. Ego Assessment

Basically, Andy seemed well-endowed, and all his ego functions (intelligence, memory, perception, language, etc.) appeared to be intact and well developed. This was evident in the general good functioning described earlier.

Open distress and anxiety are prominent current features, and in these circumscribed areas, it is clear that Andy does not have effective ego defenses in operation. He is in open conflict with his aggressive drives. His ego has difficulty dealing with the intensity of his aggression, and there are many aggressive breakthroughs at home. These breakthroughs cause him distress and anxiety and lead to many superego problems. It is important to point out that the problems in ego coping have a confined locus—in his home and with family.

It is difficult to find prominent effective defenses in these areas. The material suggests that Andy is using *regression* as a defensive operation—remaining a little boy at the anal period of development in order to ward off the sexuality and interests of an oedipal youngster. This is particularly evident in the nature of his object tie with his mother. There is some use of the mechanism of *passive into active*—earlier the material suggested that he feared separation and loss of "Mommy," but in the recent presentation he discusses *his* wish to move away and live with his neighbors. He appears to fear being abandoned and takes the active stance of abandoning his family in order to cope with the underlying anxiety.

III. Superego Assessment

Superego issues appear to be prominent in Andy's current struggles. His conscience is in the process of becoming internalized—although Andy clearly strikes out repeatedly, he seems to be experiencing a great deal of guilt over his behavior.

Andy has a severe and condemning superego. He feels he is the "worst boy" and should go to "H." His frightening dreams suggest that they are punishment dreams—a child's conscience will often punish him at night for unacceptable daytime behaviors. Moreover, in Andy's sessions, he appears to live out the role of a driven, bad "crook" who should get increasingly severe punishments by the judge (conscience).

The sources of Andy's internal distress appear, in part, to be his own reaction to his aggressive behavior toward his mother and sister. But there is also some evidence that his mother finds the "rambunctiousness" of boys distressing and therefore subtly establishes many standards of disapproval.

Andy's superego problems seem to be activated by two sources. The problems with his aggression are manifestly evident, but the material also suggests that his sexual wishes (not evident) are a source of internal concern.

Andy's conscience promotes the affects of anxiety, open distress, and guilt. Andy can become self-depreciative (he is the "worst boy"), and feelings of worthlessness also seem to be emerging. Therefore, when these conflicts are active, Andy experiences a loss of self-esteem.

The superego problems related to aggression have to be seen in context. The problems that Andy presents are circumscribed and do not affect his general behavior outside the home. The intense guilt regarding his aggressive feelings toward family members is not carried over into other areas. Andy is appropriately aggressive and competitive with peers. Teachers find him consistently happy, confident, and energetic.

IV. Genetic–Dynamic Formulation

According to the history, some problems began during the toddler period when mother (and possibly father) began to react to an energetic "rambunctious" youngster. (This was not the original perception of the parents, who pinpointed difficulties later in development.) This tension during the anal phase stimulated excessive aggression, expressed in defiant, stubborn behavior toward mother. At age 3, there was further family tension that the parents describe. Some was due to financial stress resulting from Mr. B's problems at work. Andy's sister was born and, as a troubled infant, absorbed a great deal of energy and caring. I can speculate that Andy experienced this as loss and rejection, and there was an exacerbation of his feelings of rage toward both sister and mother. Because of his aggression, he developed fears of separation and dreams of "losing Mommy," which were early imagined punishments.

Currently, Andy enters the oedipal phase of development carrying the burden of earlier problems—namely, excessive aggressivized affects unresolved from the anal period. He appears to be on the "cusp" of the oedipal period. Although the phallic development characteristic of this phase is evident, there is a lack of oedipal features that would normally unfold. What has inhibited their emergence? It appears that Andy's aggression and projected punishments for his aggression have made it difficult to enter the oedipal phase. For example, the excessive aggressivized feelings would be projected (put outside of himself) and Andy would be frightened of imagined severe punishments for transgressions. Thus, as an oedipal child, if he imagined "stealing" his mother from his father, his castration anxiety (retribution) would be very intense, causing a retreat from the sexualized wishes. The aggressivized affect state of the earlier phases often makes it more difficult for youngsters to tolerate the natural castration anxiety that emerges in the oedipal period. It appears that Andy uses regression to avoid the conflicts of this phase. Similar severe imagined punishments would emerge from rivalrous feelings with father (e.g., who is stronger, bigger, etc.). This would explain Andy's need to repress and inhibit the oedipal conflicts of this period.

In addition, both parents (mother in particular) have some difficulties with the phallic qualities of their son. The mother expressed discomfort with the noise, aggression, and boisterousness of her son and felt much greater comfort with the feminine activities of her daughter. Although Andy has some difficulties with the internal sources of his drives, it is clear that external sources also promote conflict (being acceptable to his parents regarding his sexuality and aggression).

Throughout this formulation, the circumscribed nature of Andy's difficulties has been stressed. It speaks to Andy's strength that his conflicts have not spread beyond his home and that he functions well at school and in the community. Children who contain their problems in this way suggest a diagnosis of neurosis rather than a more disturbed profile. Many areas of Andy's life were developing well.

V. Treatment Recommendations

Twice-weekly insight-oriented psychotherapy was recommended for Andy to help him deal with his internal conflicts. Andy had many strengths that would be helpful in treatment. His ego functions were intact (language, perception, memory, etc.), and he was an intelligent young man. He had a capacity for imaginative play (the crook and judge play), and he related comfortably to the therapist during the evaluation. It appeared that Andy had the capability to "play out" his internal struggles in a symbolic form, using the media in the office. His comfort with the therapist indicated that he had developed positive object relations capacities of trust, despite some of his conflicts with the grown-ups at home. These qualities would bode well for insight-oriented treatment.

Weekly sessions with the parents were also recommended. Part of the purpose of these sessions would be to help them become more empathic with Andy's internal struggles. This would emerge from discussing aspects of his history (e.g., the crisis at age 3, intense sibling rivalry, etc.). This aspect of the parent work would be a form of "parent guidance" (see Part II). Helping parents develop empathy is often a critical goal of the treatment process. For example, Andy's parents were very anxious and self-blaming when they observed Andy's manifestations of low self-esteem. Is this evidence that they failed as parents? they asked themselves. When they could come to appreciate that Andy would naturally feel guilty (worst boy) about Mary and his mother, Andy's self-berating becomes an understandable psychological process and somewhat tempers their anxiety about him. In addition, in these weekly sessions—a form of "treatment of the parent–child relationship" (see Part II)—it may be helpful to explore some of the mother's overexpectations of her children, based on her own values emerging from her family of origin, as well as the roots of her difficulties with boyish development.

Feedback Interview. Andy and his parents came for the session. I saw the parents first, while Andy stayed (drawing pictures) in the waiting room.

I told the parents that Andy was having a lot of distress with his feelings of rage. At this point we could trace some of his aggressive problems to his general intense energy level of early childhood and the discomfort his parents had with these behaviors. There also was greater tension in the family around the time of the birth of his sister. Andy appears to have felt (and continues to feel) rejected, left out, and the focus of his rage is his sister and mother. He needs to find new ways to express these strong feelings—play therapy can be a very important vehicle for sharing these feelings in a more organized way, and the goal would be to eventually help him put these feelings into words. Andy also feels terrible about having these destructive feelings. If he can find new ways to express them, we can have an opportunity to "normalize" these feelings. Right now he seems to feel as though he doesn't belong on earth (he should be in "H").

I had a number of purposes in the feedback interview. I not only wanted to give the parents an understanding of the problems, but also some sense of how child therapy works. Thus, I said, "Andy needs to find new ways to express these strong feelings (rage)." It is important to convey to parents that in child work there is typically a progression from the raw affects the child has, to play expression of these affects and, finally, to direct verbalization of these affects. The play therapy process is designed to facilitate this unfolding.

I also discussed the fact that Andy appeared stuck, and that some of the typical issues boys evidence and deal with at his age have not emerged. Boys of Andy's age naturally develop some sexy feelings and interest and also become quite competitive with their dads. I outlined two possible sources for his fear of growth. I felt that Andy's anger problem might be holding him back, and I also felt that the family may be finding the sexual, rambunctious boy hard to handle. I suggested the treatment program outlined earlier.

In this session, I wanted to establish a developmental goal, so that the parents could embrace the need for Andy to express and experience the oedipal phase of development. As the parents presented Andy's problems, they had little idea that Andy was "stuck," and the feedback session was used to develop their awareness of Andy's fear of growth.

The parents reacted by acknowledging their difficulties with Andy's intensity. Both affirmed that they come from quiet families and were unused to the kind of noise and clamor emerging from a child like Andy. His mother added that she didn't know how to handle sexual issues when they came up. Andy didn't ask questions—he might look at her breasts or want to look up her skirt. She didn't know what to do.

The parents felt they could not afford the cost of the three sessions per week, and we agreed to try meeting twice weekly with Andy and every other week with the parents.

It was also essential that I outline the work I thought I needed to do directly with the parents. Their attitudes about masculinity served as an inhibiting force in Andy's development. Often this kind of direct confrontation is avoided by the evaluator because of fears of parental discomfort and flight. In this session, the parents seemed to resonate to my conceptualizations, but one could anticipate a natural ambivalence. Was this expressed by their wish, on the one hand, to begin therapy tempered by cutting the frequency in half?

In my feedback meeting with Andy, I told him that he showed me he had a lot of worries—he felt as though he were a very bad boy—and this came from the strong mad feelings he had every day. We would be meeting once a week, and he could show me these things in his play. I could see he was a very good player already. Andy responded by wanting to immediately go back to his Lego (crook and judge) game, and I suggested that we start again next week.

Treatment Implications

Having a thorough diagnostic appraisal sets the stage for the treatment process. It orients the therapist to the future work, gives a firm foundation on which to organize the avalanche of material that will unfold, and helps him or her to be aware of material that may be missing. It is specifically helpful in (1) establishing the treatment *goals*, (2) anticipating *resistances*, and (3) anticipating some of the forms of *transference* that will emerge (see Chapter 3). These issues, as they relate to Andy, are considered more specifically before treatment is discussed.

Treatment Goals

A number of aspects of Andy's instinctual life are very troubling to him. A major goal will be to bring his pre-oedipal aggression into play form (as discussed earlier) and help him find and develop an emotional vocabulary to express his rage. When powerful aspects are verbalized, Andy's rational capacities (ego) can appraise these feelings with the help of the therapist. Second, he appears very troubled by sexual interests and curiosity (this is notable because of its marked omission), and a goal of the therapy will be to stimulate its emergence and exploration (both in therapy and in his real world). If

Andy cannot become more comfortable with sexuality during this stage of development, this bodes poorly for his comfort with his sexual feelings in adolescence and adulthood.

Another major goal that emerged is to modify his severe and attacking superego owing primarily to his unacceptable aggressive impulses. A task in the treatment will be to help him understand the natural sources of his aggression and therefore provide a human and acceptable context for the development of his rage. For example, if Andy, in the course of his treatment, can come to hear that "all kids get very angry with their sisters because they feel sisters take their mommies away," this normalizing remark from an authority can begin to modify his strong self-condemnation.

The general appraisal also allows us to set some goals in the parent work. At this point, without fully understanding the parents' discomfort with sexuality, I sense that their prohibitions may be constricting their son's development. This conceptualization provides a direction for the work with the parents—namely, to explore their own feelings about childhood sexuality and to normalize its existence in Andy.

Resistances

What kind of resistances can be expected from Andy in the treatment process? The appraisal has, in part, focused on Andy's ego—particularly in the responses he used to ward off, repress, and defend against the conscious emergence of unacceptable impulses. These ego responses (defense) will tend to emerge in the treatment hour and become the specific forms of *resistance* in the therapy. The defenses we highlighted were *repression, denial, regression,* and *passive into active.* How might they emerge as resistances?

Consider one defense process as an example—regression. On the basis of the diagnostic understanding, I would anticipate that Andy's sadistic play in the therapy sessions would have a number of uses. One would be to express his rage, but another purpose would be a form of resistance—the use of the defense of *regression.* Andy's sadistic behavior keeps him as the younger anal child, and away from the sexual, oedipal feelings of a boy his age. With the understanding of the nature of his typical resistance (defense), I can anticipate an interpretative direction. "Often guys need to beat up their mommies all the time (my response to anticipated play in the treatment hour), because it can be very scary to show their strong caring feelings." This form of defense (resistance) interpretation can slowly allow the child to become aware of his underlying impulses. Often this kind of interpretation helps the child to bring out the affects that have been surpressed.

Transference

The diagnostic appraisal can also help to prepare the therapist for the forms of transferences that will emerge. All patients live out their feelings and experiences within the treatment, and the history gathered provides a road map of potential scenarios.

On one level, I can anticipate that Andy will come to develop a father transference—that some of the forbidden and frightening aspects of the oedipal rivalry will emerge. In fact, it would not be unusual for them to emerge in treatment rather than at home, inasmuch as there is often a feeling of relative safety in the therapy situation.

The area of sibling rivalry has been a striking issue in Andy's life. How might these affects emerge in the treatment hour? I anticipate that Andy will express strong feelings about the "siblings" in the office—my other child patients. Although they are not there directly, evidence of their existence is everywhere. How will Andy react to the other childrens' drawings that he sees in the office, to the private drawers that house their work (each child patient has a private drawer), to the general toys that he has to share with the patient/siblings? In these areas, Andy is likely to live out the affects he experiences toward Mary, *transferring* into the treatment the conflicts he experiences at home.

Although we clearly cannot anticipate all the goals, resistances, and transferences, the diagnostic appraisal provides a critical context for the evolving treatment material. Returning again and again to the diagnostic framework, reformulating and reshaping our original ideas, gives shape to the treatment strategy and the interventions that we develop.

Conclusion

I cannot emphasize enough the need for a thorough and comprehensive evaluation before one embarks on treatment. There is currently enormous pressure to shorten the evaluation process, and the pressure is primarily from third-party insurance carriers. Many practitioners in the mental health field find rationalizations and submit to the mandate for truncated evaluations. A systematic evaluation provides the therapist with a general outline for the case and a strategy for the work. It places the therapist's feet solidly on the ground.

Many clinical issues are understood when we refer back to our earliest appraisal. For example, a natural problem in our work is our countertransference reactions to child and parents. We often need to temper our immediate (or intuitive) reactions. Suppose, for example, that Andy destroys another child's creations in the office. Although I would need to stop him, my understanding that he was expressing a sibling transference would temper my reaction and help me phrase a helpful verbal intervention. This kind of understanding can only come from the diagnostic appraisal. The diagnostic workup is a source of self-supervision and self-consultation, the foundation to which one needs to refer again and again.

Because the evaluation is the backbone of the case, I invariably write up a case after a completed appraisal, using the structure outlined in this chapter. This is a 4-to-5-hour exercise—writing up both the descriptive material and the formulation. This is an excercise that illuminates the case, raises questions that must be further explored, and provides direction and insight. I write out this evaluation before my feedback session, and the ideas form the basis for my feedback discussion. This evaluation is the start of my file in each case.

THE FIRST 4 MONTHS

The structure for the therapy with Andy began to evolve in the evaluation sessions. Andy immediately took to the toys that were available and began to play. As noted earlier, *play is the emotional language of children, and it is through their play that they will bring forth their fantasy, affective life.* Child therapists must provide the equipment (toys) that the child can use for his projections, and then essentially *get out of the way* and allow this internal world to unfold. My initial involvement with Andy was to ask some questions about his play, not deciding or directing it, so that I could understand the story that he wanted to develop. It is the child, not the therapist, who sets the play agenda.

The therapeutic structure must also be a safe one, and this is often established through small actions and prohibitions. If the child is using a crayon and he wants to tear off the wrapper, I might suggest that he just take off enough so that the end of the crayon is exposed and useful. Or if a "play karate chop" looks as thought it can break one of the wooden slats of the Lincoln Logs, I will caution him about the amount of force he can use. These small, continuous limits establish a boundary for most children. The child can play out and act out all sorts of aggressive or sexual ideas, but the force of the play cannot damage or break things in reality. This is a relieving boundary for the child, when he is given permission to explore his internal life.

Slowly, over the first few sessions (evaluation and therapy), I outline with the child what we will be doing together and the format of the work. I highlight the child's worries—in this case, I discussed with Andy that he felt that he was a bad boy, and this came from his strong, everyday mad feelings. I told him that I am a worry doctor who helps boys with these feelings. These worries come from inside feelings, from our inside imagination. And Andy was already showing me some of these feelings in his play. In fact, play is our work. These ideas are not discussed in one paragraph, as they are here, but emerge slowly over the first four to five sessions. Thus, I begin to define in the child's language, our mission (to help him with his worries), who I am (a worry doctor), and the format of our work (the use of play, which we will attempt to develop and understand together).

Early Play Sessions with Andy

Andy continues the same game of the crook-police-judge using his Legos. The crook is jailed for stealing, only to escape, and he receives greater and greater punishments. He is chased by the police, who eventually capture him again, and the police now use radar to find him. The play begins to get more intense and gory. When the police surround the crook, they bring out trucks, jeeps, and other such equipment. They begin running over the crook in their rage, reacting to his repeated crimes. I imitate Andy's play—I take on the role of the terrified crook, scared about what is happening. "No, no, don't run me over," I say, in a falsetto voice. "Help, you're hurting me," I express in the play. Andy gleefully does his dirty work. The head comes off, the legs of the criminal come off. Blood pops out of the torso. I put words to the attack—"The head is popping off . . . blood is shooting out of his body," and so forth. I can see the sadism and cruelty emerge, and Andy is entranced by the game.

Then Andy puts the dismembered crook back together, and places him in jail. But he escapes again, and the torturing experience is repeated, with my involvement. I continue to both describe the tortures and act the role of the hurt crook-victim. I also begin to make some additional comments during this activity. "Boy, this guy is getting 'smutched'". "Here go those 'smutch' feelings again." "This story has a lot of 'smutch' action." The word "smutch" is my metaphor for smashing, sadistic feelings. These comments are not delivered in a play voice, but in the therapist's natural observing ego voice. At the end of each hour, we clean up together. We decide which Lego constructions that Andy made we will keep in his private drawer (e.g., the police helicopter) for the continued game, and which toys (trucks, jeeps) will be returned for general use.

A major treatment goal is to help Andy deal with his rage and sadism. Therefore, one would expect these affects to appear in his play, and an initial goal would be to highlight these elements and put words to them. This is an enormous opportunity. These are the feelings that Andy wishes to disown and that cause his conscience to plague him. The harsh punishments for the crook are the initial expressions of Andy's sadism. In the play sequences, with me as a player, Andy elaborates the torture and mayhem that express his sadism and rage. (In this case, they come out in superego form—as severe punishments for transgressions. He has a severe, punishing superego, which is fueled by his aggressive drives.) Andy begins to express and elaborate these troubling affects, which cause him intense distress. As I join his play, I implicitly provide him permission to express these feelings.

I bring in the terms "smutch" and "smutch feelings." The reason for my using this word and phrase is to establish a metaphor that we can use together. Andy "smutches" the crook, as he runs him over in the play. He smashes the crook. The smutch activity is his sadistic activity. When this metaphor becomes established, it comes to symbolize Andy's sadistic feelings. This is a phenomenon that we can look at and discuss together. The "smutch" word will come to stand, generally, for Andy's internal rage in many circumstances. Technically, I am introducing a "confrontation" (see the introduction to Part III), an intervention in which the phenomenon I feel we should work on is made explicit to the patient's ego. This is a first step, and we need some time to establish that Andy indeed has smutch (sadistic) feelings. After we establish that these feelings exist within him, we can later go on to learn what stimulates such feelings and at whom they are directed. "Smutch" is also a playful word, the kind of word that would attract a 5-or-6-year-old, and it doesn't carry the pejorative tone of words like "angry feeling" or "rageful feelings." It is critical to develop this special vocabulary with children that highlights both a nonjudgmental attitude and an ability to enter the world of the child.

During these initial hours, Andy interspersed other activities with instances of crook-police-judge play. He showed me recent karate kicks he had learned, and when he demonstrated how high he could kick, he accompanied each thrust with a gutteral "Hyaa." He also established a basketball game (using a hoop and a Nerf ball I have available—the hoop fits on the door), in which he shoots and scores and I keep score of his achievements. His intent was to rack up a huge score (e.g., 30 points), which I was required to record on a score sheet, and this accomplishment was retained for his private drawer. Each hour he would review his past attainment, and seek to set a new record. A score of 40 points was deposited in his drawer in a subsequent hour, and Andy was proud.

An important role in child psychotherapy is the functioning of the therapist as a "developmental facilitator." (See Chapter 1.) The child is in the process of development, and the therapist must also deal with the manifestations and stresses of normal development that emerges. The child patient is rapidly changing as he grows: His ego is expanding, his drives are unfolding, he establishes new identities, his consciousness and self-consciousness are developing. The therapist is in a central position to be instrumental in this developmental process. In child work, the therapist is therefore not only dealing with the conflicts the child has developed, but also becomes an important new object for approval and identification.

In the preceding clinical material, Andy expresses a natural need for the approval of his emerging phallic behavior. Karate kicks and high basketball scores mean he is an emerging powerful, strong, competitive boy. He specifically seeks (and receives) my approval and admiration for his male accomplishments, and this aspect of my work with Andy is part of the developmental facilitation role of a therapist. In Andy's family, the expression of these affects meet troubling and anxious responses; they become part of the focus of the parent work in the course of the treatment, which I will describe later.

Andy continues the crook-smutch play as the centerpiece of the early hours during the first 20 sessions. The jail format—escape, stealing, capture—continues, and the crook is smutched mightily. The crook now carries a hidden, sneaky gun, so there is more of a battle with his capture. He enjoys how I vivify the thief's pain as he sadistically kills and dismembers. And he grinds and pounds clay into the tortured crook. Therefore, our cleanup session takes longer, as we have to clean up the clay-splattered Lego pieces.

I am now adding to my comments during these hours. I comment that all boys have smutching (sadistic) feelings. I discuss all of the people that Andy would like to smutch sometimes. Sometimes upsetting things happen at home, and he must feel like smutching his sister, mother, or father. These ideas come from my understanding of Andy's history. During one such soliloquy, Andy tells me again that he steals candy from his sister's room. I note that maybe he worries that he will be taken to a big judge, and that terrible things will happen to him.

Other activities of the hours include telling me about kindergarten. He likes his teacher, Mrs. C, and he can print his name (which he exhibits). He gets carried away, tells me he can write "in cursive," and proceeds to scribble. I playfully admire his attempt at cursive writing, which he tells me no one else in his class can do.

In the vein of his phallic prowess, he develops an airplane game. Together we make paper airplanes, that can fly across the room. In the game format, I fly my planes across the room. His planes are missiles, and he flies them to shoot me down in midair. Chethik, the new object, enhances his growing masculinity.

In these sessions, I take the smutch feelings one step further. I link them to the idea that all boys have smutch feelings against close members of the family when they become frustrated. This is a preparation process for later interpretations and reconstructions about why Andy developed his troubling, sadistic feelings. My comments continue to be interventions that are part of the preparation process—they are confrontations *and* clarifications *(interventions that are preconscious), and I am again focusing on this aspect of the play to highlight its importance in our work. (See the introduction to Part III.) Andy is aware that he has this kind of rage toward his mother and sister, although he does not like to dwell on these feelings.*

In this period, I am in the pre-insight phase of my work with this youngster. I am introducing and highlighting his sadistic feelings and the objects of his sadistic feelings. Andy needs a period to become

*somewhat comfortable with the idea that we can put his precon-
scious feelings into words, and that this aspect of his feeling life will
be an important part of our work.*

*Toward the end of these 20 sessions, I suggested we make a spe-
cial book, called the Smutch Book. (This is a plain manila folder, on
which I print out this title.) Andy takes clay and adds to the cover by
"smutching" a large clay stain on the folder. I print comments or
draw pictures on drawing paper to summarize some of the ideas of
the hour, and place these sheets into the folder. I write that all boys
have smutching feelings (also using his idea of the symbolic clay
stain), and I draw a picture of a mom, dad, and sister, indicating dia-
grammatically how angry smutch feelings can come their way. Now,
at the start of each session, I take out the Smutch Book and place it
in the background, indicating by this action that we may have something to enter in it later in the session. It is important, in work with
pre-odeipal, oedipal, and latency children, to concretize aspects of
the work together. The Smutch Book tangibly holds some of the
ideas that are discussed together over a period of time. Thus, with
other children one might develop a Divorce Book or a Blowup Book,
depending on the important themes of the treatment. With some children who have been severely traumatized in the past (e.g., because of
sexual abuse), I have developed a Scary Time Book, in which we
slowly piece together some aspects of a past event that have disturbed the child's functioning. Because all children in treatment
struggle with sexual developmental issues, I typically develop a Body
Book as well, in which ideas about sexuality are noted. In the course
of therapy I usually develop two to four "theme books" with the
child.*

*Although Andy enjoys the play and enjoys having the therapist
as a player, he feels uncomfortable and becomes anxious as I comment on the play or develop the Smutch Book. Andy has, like all children, an immature therapeutic alliance. He may come to like the
therapist and become attached to the therapist (a libidinal tie), but he
does not identify with the goals of the treatment, which are to find
new ways to express and accept aspects of his aggressive drive. The
rational goals of the treatment, as a foundation for the mature aspects of an alliance, are developed with adult patients. Children have
little capacity to observe themselves, or to tolerate psychic pain, and
therefore have little internal motivation for the psychotherapy pro-*
cess. (For a fuller discussion, see Chapter 1.)

The books we develop together contain some self-examination and summarize our thinking about his problems. Andy often doesn't really want to use the Smutch Book, though he may comply with the therapist's use of the book. Just as Andy does not necessarily "want" math and language arts periods in school but participates in the school day, so he participates in the treatment hour.

Early Work with Parents

As noted earlier, in the feedback session with the parents I outlined some of the internal problems that Andy had with both aggression and sexuality, and I also indicated the parents' own discomfort with Andy's emerging rough boyishness. In this early period, the parents seemed very positive and eager to work together with me. They described some changes at home involving Andy and their responses to him.

The parents report that when treatment began, play broke out at home. Andy began playing "Bear" at home, and Bear was a bad character. Bear stole cars and jewelry and was sent to jail. The parents said that Andy made it clear that he was Bear, and he also showed them how Bear did karate.

The parents also reported that Andy's harassment of his younger sister continued unremittingly. For example, he shoots her with a gun, openly wishing she were dead. When he does this, in his intense way, the play is very distressing to his sister. His father noted in the parent session that he felt he could be helpful to Andy by pointing out that sometimes brothers hate sisters. Mother also noted that she now sees that sometimes Mary starts some of their difficulties. She hits or teases Andy, and she is also capable of having tantrums of her own.

The parents said that they are were experiencing increasing relief because they felt that they had some perspective and understanding of Andy's behavior. The mother stated that for a considerable period she felt intensely angry toward Andy, and hated and felt ashamed at having that kind of reaction to her child. Father said that when Andy was on an "I hate Mary" jag one day, he explained to him that they always wanted to have a family of four—the parents, a boy, and a girl. Both parents felt that since treatment began, it was easier to talk directly to Andy.

I felt, in this situation, that the family as a whole was experiencing a great deal of relief because of the evaluation and the early treatment process. An important ingredient of this relief was the per-

spective that the therapist was providing. Andy was not seen as disturbed, as the parents had feared. The explanations for his behavior (e.g., jealousy) seemed to provide an acceptable and understandable context for their son's aggression and anxiety.

The parents reported that when treatment began, "play broke out at home." This was important, because the parents had noted earlier that Andy had lost his playfulness. Play adaptively allows for all sorts of affects to be expressed and discharged. Was Andy now able to play again because this form of expression was encouraged in his sessions? Or could he now play at home because his parents were more comfortable with instinctualized play expression, as a result of the therapist's explanations? I felt that both factors were at work.

The parents want to be helpful and make use of their new understanding. Father notes to Andy that "brothers hate sisters sometimes," beginning to sanction Andy's underlying feelings that were previously very troubling to the parents. It is interesting to note that in these early sessions, Andy is not the only villain. Suddenly mother sees that Mary can provoke her brother and create some of the sibling tension. I felt the parents experienced relief because of their growing understanding, and a conviction that this new process (including the work with the parents) would promote change. This change began immediately and accelerated in this 4-month period.

It is not unusual that changes can occur quickly in families because of the new developmental context that a child therapist can provide. This does not mean that early symptom relief (in this case there was some change in the first few months) will be sustained. Unfortunately, with the current pressure for short-term work and insurance funding limitations, the early and transitory blossoming that can accompany the commencing of treatment is seen as evidence that termination is warranted. Although Andy experiences some relief, the underlying sources of the troubling sadistic/sexual fantasies have not emerged nor been explored.

After a period of about 2 months, the parents began to discover that their children were indeed interested in sexuality. Words like "bosom," "tushie," "dick," and "weiner" came up in giggling discussions between the children at mealtimes or in the bathroom. Mary used as many words as Andy, the parents observed. Feeling supported by the therapy, the parents began to educate the children. They taught the children the correct words for the parts of the body but also allowed them to use their "natural" words. They bought several cartoon-like books about sexuality to keep in the home and checked out their suitability with the therapist. This became an engaging project for the family, and they had a sense of pride in the process.

The parents noted that as they began to discuss the body, natural questions emerged from Andy about the functions of the various body parts. "Why do mommies have breasts?" "Why does my penis get stiff?" Eventually, the father described the sexual act to Andy—how the penis of the daddy goes into the vagina of the mother—and he found that Andy wanted this described over and over again. Andy said, "I love it," as if this revelation led to a sense of discovery. He asked whether his parents did this. He wanted to know whether you make a baby each time. Andy "confessed" to his father that he thought about naked ladies, and his father commented supportively that all men thought about ladies.

Toward the end of this 4-month period (early work), the parents found Andy very troubled for several days. He became more fearful—he was afraid to be in his bedroom at night. For several nights, he wet his bed. For the first time, Andy found a way to describe his trouble in words. He finally told his parents that a neighborhood bully was attacking him on the school bus, sitting on him and punching him. The parents were able to help Andy find a solution—to talk with the bus driver, who kept Andy near the front of the bus, in closer observation. They all felt relieved with the way this problem worked out, and Andy's acute symptomatic behavior disappeared.

I felt there was further evidence of the parents' identification with the goals of the treatment in these sessions. Picking up on my earlier explanation of Andy's developmental anxieties about sexuality, the parents attempted to introduce this topic and bring up the world of sexuality. I was unsure about how internally comfortable the parents were with this topic, but they forged ahead. They recognized Andy's intense interest and need for understanding. and gained a good sense of their own competence as they helped their son.

There were many areas of better communication between Andy and his parents in this early period. They could be more empathic and comforting when he evidenced stress, and Andy responded with new comfort in their relationship. He found a way to put into words his peer distress (the bully incident), and they helped him find a solution.

Why were the parents responding so constructively at this point? Clearly, they were highly invested in functioning as good and effec-

*tive parents. The emotional problems Andy was developing had at-
tacked their faith in their parenting abilities. In this situation, my explanations of Andy's difficulties (including their role in the problems)
did not produce an overwhelming narcissistic injury. Rather, it mobilized them to become active, and as they saw evidence of their effectiveness, it seemed to begin to restore their sense of efficacy in this
stage of parenthood.*

THE MIDDLE PHASE

In the early period of my work with Andy, he introduced his
aggressive–sadistic affects expressed in the crook and police play,
and we developed the metaphor of Andy's "smutch feeling" to embrace these affects. I also introduced the idea that all boys had these
smutch feelings at times, toward moms, dads and sisters. Therefore,
not only did he have sadistic feelings, but these were objects against
whom he directed his rage. This theme continued in the middle phase
of our work.

In this new period, Andy began to use a different medium in
play—he began to draw. In his wish to be praised and receive my approval, he sought to develop drawings that could be valued and exhibited on my bulletin board.

The bulletin board is part of the setting where the therapy takes
place. It is enormously helpful to think of the therapist and the setting of the treatment as having the potential to facilitate transference.
By transference, I mean that current intense issues within the family
will be lived out within the four walls of the treatment space. Many
natural issues emerge in reaction to the bulletin board, the reserved
wall space for display of the patients' drawings. For example, if I currently have four children in treatment, I reserve one-fourth of the
wall space for each child. Children often react to the amount of space
they are accorded. Am I getting my fair share, they wonder? Sometimes they want to put up extra pictures to claim more of the space
than the others. They compare the quality of their drawings. They
seem to be asking, "Is my drawing better than the others?" "Do I
have more talent?" "Whom do you like best?" The bulletin board
therefore becomes a vast repository for displaced sibling issues. The
immediate displaced siblings are the other unseen patients in my
care, but these new siblings will evoke all the feelings a patient has

about his real-life brothers and sisters. The therapist will potentially become the approving or withholding parent. Thus, the apparently simple act of displaying a drawing can elicit many intense issues of the family transference currently in play at home. These issues are evoked not only by the bulletin board, but also by toy usage, private drawers, and the like. Andy, in the following material, reacts strongly to his unseen competitive siblings.

Play Sessions with Andy

Andy drew pictures and, at my behest, developed stories about his drawings. I commented that drawings and stories come from his imagination and that they are a very good way of telling us about his inside feelings. I wrote his stories as they emerged, and we would attach the commentary to his drawings. Thus, I could record them with animation, have him elaborate on some themes, and have an opportunity to comment on the issues he was developing—as I did with the shark epidsode.

Andy developed his shark drawing over several sessions, and he definitely wanted this prize creation hung on the wall (see Figure 11.1). He dictated the following intense story with affect: "We see a lot of ground and water and sun. In the sea there are SHARKS who can bite you. The big sharks have real big teeth. The sharks are eating all of the little fish. They don't like the little fish swimming in the shark's place. LOOK, WE CAN SEE THE BLOOD. Another little fish is bitten, and we can see all of the b-l-o-o-d come out, and more and more blood. Uh oh, another fish is caught."

I commented, after reading his story to him, that those sharks have a lot of "smutch-biting" feelings, and that they certainly didn't want those little fish to be living anywhere near them in this part of the sea. Boys also get smutch feelings at the little fish who are swimming around in their house. Although Andy showed no visible response for a few minutes, he suddenly fashioned a little girl out of clay and had her swimming in the water. The stapler on the play table became the shark mouth, and the girl screamed as the shark chewed off the arms and legs and little girl's head. I said that I could see he had very strong smutch feelings, and that all boys feel strong hating feelings toward their little sisters at times.

Toward the end of the session, Andy definitely wanted this picture hung. I use pushpins to hang the drawings, and Andy himself wanted to use these sharp pins, which I allowed. When he came near an adjacent drawing (from a gifted young artist patient) he suddenly stabbed this creation several times with his sharp pushpin. His face evidenced rage. I

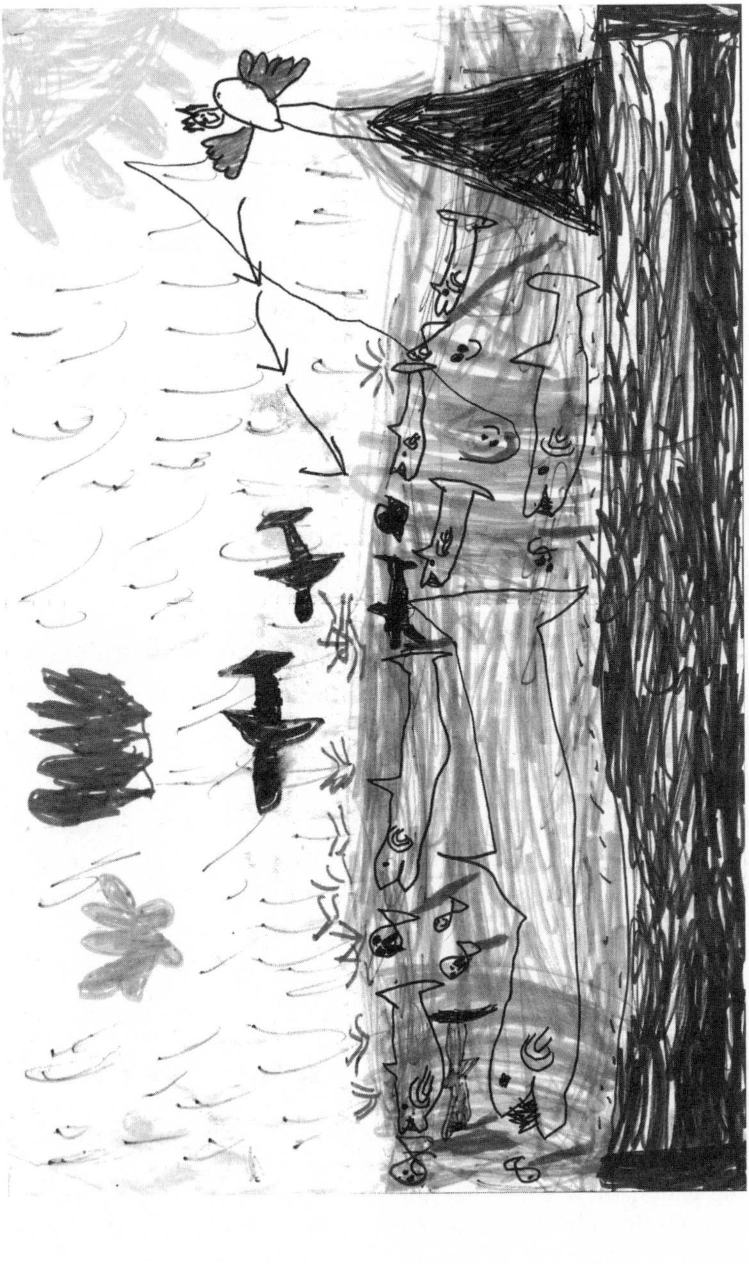

FIGURE 11.1. Andy's shark drawing.

stopped Andy, and there was no permanent damage to the drawing. I said that he couldn't tear other people's pictures, but I could see that, just as at home, he wanted to be my special fish and the only one in my office. I added that the other people I see make him feel very jealous, just as Mary does at home. When boys are little, I said, they feel very special, but when a little Mary is born and comes home from the hospital, they can feel very thrown out.

The inference I made from his drawing was that Andy was the sadistic shark, who was delighting in bloodying the smaller fish, his sibling. The sea was like his crowded home filled with siblings; he was the killer who hated the small intruders. I used these ideas in my comments to him during the hour. Andy responded and confirmed my interpretation, the stapler-shark play further expressing these rageful affects. Later in the hour he reexperienced these feelings in the transference, by attacking the drawing of another sibling/patient. Thus, he lived out his conflicts at home and, simultaneously, in the office.

During this hour there was an important new element. I had an opportunity to make an interpretation leading to insight. Insight occurs when intensely experienced affects and some understanding of these affects come together. Andy was aware of his intense raw rage and generally had the feeling that these affects were terrible— he was the "worst boy." In this work together, I helped him to understand what these affects are about— that he is expressing hatred toward his sister, and these affects emerge because he is very jealous that she has taken away his feelings of specialness. Thus, these raw "killer" feelings now began to have a new context, and they now had an understandable human source. Our goal was to modify Andy's harsh superego reactions toward himself and for him to take in the idea that all children have intensely jealous feelings and associated rage toward younger siblings.

The following week Andy continued to work on his shark drawing and dictated the following story: "There is a person, a boy, standing on a big rock, and he is throwing rocks in the water. He wanted to hit the sharks. He hates them because they are biting everyone. If the boy tried to swim in the water, they would bite him. Look, another fish is bitten by the sharks. The bloody fish are dead and go up to fish heaven. Uh oh, we see one safe fish. No, it is bitten and the guts come out."

In my comments, I drew attention to the boy. I told Andy the boy hates the sharks because he feels they are very bad biters. Sometimes Andy feels he is a very bad boy because of his biting feelings. Somebody should punish or hurt him—there should even be a judge who would put him in jail.

The boy in the drawing, standing above and watching the sea scene, I felt, represented Andy's watchful superego. It suggested a strong internal conflict—his biting aggression draws a harsh counter-reaction from his conscience. In his daily existence we see both the expressions of his direct rage and the accompanying self-hatred. My interventions are attempts to connect his self-attack (his low self-esteem) to his aggression and to make him aware that what all children naturally experience is somehow unacceptable to him.

Andy put the finishing touches on his shark drawing and dictated an ending chapter to his story. "Guess what? The boy finally liked the sharks, and said, 'I'm sorry I threw a rock at you!' The sharks said they would let the boy swim in the water, and he did. The boy got a fishing pole. The fish ate his worm and had a nice meal, and then the boy caught the fish. He said "'Thank you' to the sharks, and they said 'You are welcome'." I commented on how polite and good everyone had become. I noted that I thought that Andy felt bad about all the blood and killing, so he was showing me that everyone was very, very good.

In this sequence, the last material was an attempt to defensively undo the mayhem of recent hours.

For a number of weeks Andy continued to use his drawing skills, drawing many witches, which highlighted his aggression toward his mother and his fears of his "mean mommie" attacking him. I had an opportunity to discuss the idea that boys get very strong smutch feelings toward moms when new babies are born—they feel very "thrown out."

In his sessions, Andy wants to play school. He has me write out all the names he knows. I print out "Mom," "Dad," "Mary," and the names of friends: "Kevin," "Brian," "Chris," and so on. Next to each, Andy draws a symbol. Near his friends, he draws a star. Next to his dad, a heart emerges, but Mary gets the shark's mouth and his mother has a dagger near her name. I comment Mother and Mary get all the smutch feelings he has.

Andy moves to the playhouse. It is dark, at night, and a boy named Michael (he tells me) is trying to go to sleep. Andy makes ghost sounds coming from the second floor, and Michael is considering walking up into the dark. (In the enactment, I play out some scary feelings in identification with Michael.) The sounds are frightening, Michael is scared, and then we even hear footsteps—heavy, pounding footsteps. Michael goes up slowly, and FRANKENSTEIN is there. (He uses a larger male doll.) And Frankenstein is there with mother and Mary. Michael watches as Frankenstein kills Mary and Mother. Particularly crushing blows seem to befall the mother.

I comment that I know that Andy has a lot of Frankenstein monster feelings inside of him. Andy was very angry when his sister came home. His mother then spent a lot of time with Mary, and it felt as though she went away from him and gave everything to Mary. Boys get upset and sad and very, very angry.

The Michael play went on for a number of sessions, with very similar scenarios. After some of this work, the parents reported that Andy was less fearful of the dark, less fearful of going upstairs to his bedroom or to the basement or attic. These "hidden" areas were becoming less frightening.

In this period of play the sibling issues continue, and there is a greater opportunity to focus on Andy's rage toward his mother as well as Mary. The play allows the therapist to provide further insight. Andy fears the monsters that are in the dark corners of his home—they will do mayhem, so he tends to stay on the well-lit, homey first floor. In his unfolding material, I have an opportunity to understand that the monsters are a projection Andy himself has a lot of monster feelings. In my comments, they emerge as natural monster feelings, because they came about when he had the intense experience of being deserted by his mother. Because there is evidence of symptom alleviation, Andy appears to be able to take in this interpretation. He becomes less frightened of the dark, the monsters and ghosts. It is as though he can accept the idea that although the outside monsters disappear, they are really within him. His sense of relief indicates further that he can allow himself these rageful feelings.

In this midphase period, Andy did a lot of work on his jealousy of sister and loss of mother and the self-punishing consequences of his aggression.

Work with Parents

For several months the parents reported a significant decrease in Andy's aggressive outbursts toward his mother and Mary and a lessening of the self-abusive behavior that had been so troubling 6 months earlier. The therapy provided new outlets for Andy for these feelings to be expressed and understood.

In one session in this period, the mother indicated that she had been withholding a memory of a dream she had when Andy was a little boy. The dream always made her feel very guilty, and she didn't understand why. The dream occurred when Andy was a toddler and was a very vigorous little boy. She recalled being exhausted by him and needing to nap when he finally took a nap in the afternoon. On one occasion, as she took this nap, she dreamt that a little dog was nipping and biting her legs. She ran from the dog and climbed a tree in order to escape him. In the current session, Mrs. B now readily interpreted the dream. Even when Andy was a toddler, she felt that he was too much for her, and she wanted to escape him. She recognized that she felt intense guilt and shame about these "getting rid of" feelings. Relating this memory had a confessional quality for Mrs. B. She was very upset about the discomfort she had with Andy's energy and level of activity. She realized, more and more as we worked together, that although Andy's temperament was an intense one, it wasn't a sign of pathology.

In the following session, Mrs. B had more memories of her childhood. There were two boys her age on her street who were terrors in the neighborhood. They were always getting into trouble and made it difficult for the defenseless girls with whom she played. These boys were obnoxious and wouldn't leave the others alone. Chris, one of the neighborhood boys, was a particular bully. She revealed how she and her friends had built a snow fort (she was 8 or 9 years old) and Chris broke it apart. She was so furious that she forgot herself, pummeled him, and, to her surprise, he cried and ran off. She recalled that Chris got into much trouble as a teenager and, she assumed, had a bad fate.

This material allowed Mrs. B to become aware that she had internally identified Andy with these bad bullies of her past. She recoiled from them (as she did with Andy), was furious with their threatening behavior, and she identified Mary as one of the defenseless girls of her old neighborhood. She currently felt, as she explored these ideas in the sessions, that these fearful images didn't fully match the present. Andy was not a loser like those youngsters had been; he had friends and did well in school, in contrast to the children of her past. And Mary was in reality no pushover who always needed her protection and vigilance.

In the earlier phase of treatment, the mode of the work with the parents had been "parent guidance." I helped the parents to understand the roots of Andy's rage and the process of his internal guilt, which promoted his low self-esteem. This helped the parents to empathize with Andy's struggles and made them less angry and frightened. In the these sessions (midphase) with the parents, the work took a significant turn. The mother began to explore her internal reactions to her child and how they were linked to her own childhood experiences. The modality of the parent work shifted into "treatment of the parent–child relationship" (For a full discussion of various aspects of parent work, see Part II.).

As Mrs. B became more comfortable with the parent work, she allowed herself to explore her internal reactions to her child, which had contributed to her emotional alienation from him. Intuitively, she felt there was an inappropriate aversion to Andy's intensity. She "confessed" that this began when he was a toddler (the dream). As she explored her associations, she had clearly linked him to the childhood troublemakers and bullies—the "bad boys" of her neighborhood. These were unconscious associations that had molded her emotional response toward her son. When these links could be discussed consciously, Mrs. B was able to separate her fears of the past from the reality of the present: Andy really did not fulfill the image of the boys of the past. This insight allowed her to begin to respond differently to Andy's behavior. Thus, the process of treatment of the parent–child relationship can help a parent deal with an unconscious fantasy about a child, without the parent having enter into his or her own personal psychotherapy.

I felt that this new awareness helped Mrs. B to respond more empathically to her son, because she could recognize her internal "childhood" reaction and correct her response. I did not feel that our work completely eliminated the sources of Mrs. B's responses to phallic behavior. Were there earlier roots? Did she have difficulty with a relationship with her brother or father? These aspects would normally be fully explored in individual psychotherapy. However, her self-exploration in the parent work allowed her to significantly modify her responses to her son.

As the mother worked on her feelings, the father said that he was "chomping at the bit." He had seen a lot of progress in Andy and wondered how much longer they would need to come. With my encouragement, he expressed his ideas that they were continuing to spend a lot of time, money, and effort, and he worried that people get addicted to therapy. When I asked more about the addiction idea, Mr. B said that Andy was usually "chomping at the bit" to come to see me. He then acknowledged his worry that Andy could come to like me too much.

I said that I felt the major reason for Andy's attachment to me was that he could bring forbidden ideas, and this provided some relief for him. I also discussed with the parents some of my original formulation. Although Andy's anger had definitely abated and he was clearly more comfortable with himself, I did not feel that his comfort extended to his sexuality. He remained too frightened of these feelings than we would want at this stage of development. I worried that his discomfort with this aspect of himself could lay a foundation for problems, in adolescence and adulthood, in being a sexual man. The parents agreed to continue, deferring to my general conception.

One has to anticipate that parents will become resistant during the course of the work. I felt there were a number of reasons that Mr. B was "chomping at the bit." He felt threatened about the tie that Andy had developed with me. Would I become the better parent? In addition, both parents were uncomfortable with the exploration of sexuality in childhood, and this promoted the hope that the therapy would already be completed.

I have found it very helpful to address parental resistance at the slightest hint of its presence. Lateness in bringing the child or paying the bill may be an indicator. In the preceding material, I was able to help the parents recommit themselves to the process because I could reiterate goals that I had originally shared with them. In the feedback session, I had outlined Andy's trepidation in entering the oedipal struggle, and said that despite the symptomatic improvement, Andy seemed to continue to remain "at the cusp" of this developmental stage. It is extremely valuable to fully outline our understanding at the start of treatment and to avoid premature termination when some symptom relief becomes evident. In our educative process with parents, it is important to help them understand that we utilize a developmental framework as the basis of our assessment, rather than a primary focus on symptoms or behavioral problems. I discussed with Andy's parents that inasmuch as he did not experience oedipal phase developmental issues, his treatment was not completed.

THE LAST TREATMENT PHASE
AND TERMINATION

Much of the material in this latter part of treatment was concerned with Andy's phallic behavior and specific sexual fantasies. He ushered in this material through his play with Legos.

Sessions with Andy

Andy carefully constructs a "jet ski" that has a special shooter on the front of it. A man rides this jet ski, and in this play the jet ski races faster and faster. The major purpose in this story is to finally have the jet ski crash, and to crash in such a way that the front shooter gets broken off. After the crash of the jet ski, the man also falls off and ends up losing an arm, leg, or head. This is repeated in pleasurable, but also anxiety-producing, play. During these enactments, Andy is also discussing some of his enthusiastic climbing—how he loves to climb on the monkey bars, and how he now gets all the way across; how he has developed new tricks on his bike. With his discussion, the jet ski continues to crash, the front shooter repeatedly comes off, and the driver loses a piece of his anatomy.

I comment that all boys who are growing up worry about their bodies. Can they get hurt? Can something come off their bodies? As I make these comments I develop a new book for us which I entitle the "Body Book" (a manila folder with the words "Body Book" in bold print) to add to the Smutch Book we have already developed. At the end of the hour I put a sheet into the book, with the heading "Body Worries." Under that I write, "Boys worry about whether something could happen to their shooters," and draw stick figures illustrating the worry.

This introduces a period where a great deal of sexual material and preoccupation emerges, and Andy often wants to add his drawings into the Body Book. First he draws a series of "Do's" and "Don'ts." He draws a boy eating a hamburger with a rock in it, then makes an anatomical drawing in which the rock gets stuck in the boy's stomach. He adds the word "Don't" at the top, with fanfare and pleasure. He writes the word "Do" when a boy eats a normal hamburger, and we trace the digestive system working smoothly. He draws a "Don't" picture of a boy eating a worm, and he giggles as he makes the boy "barf."

He then draws a series of "secret pictures." The initial one is of a naked boy with penis peeing into the toilet. He draws a picture of a girl with a vagina, also going to the toilet to pee. Other secret pictures include backsides. These are deposited into the Body Book, and the whole book is reviewed frequently. I note to Andy that all boys are very curious about naked people, all the parts of the body, and these are important topics for us to talk about (see Figure 11.2).

The inference I develop from the Lego-crashing, broken-shooter play is that Andy is living out castration anxiety, worries about bodily injury. The jet ski appears to me to be a self-representation, a little boy with many exciting, racing, sexual feelings that can lead to a flooding of excitement and bodily injury. Therefore, after a period of repeated play, I comment on the general worry boys have about their bodies and develop the Body Book with Andy. When he adds comments about his climbing activities, this confirms for me his current phallic pursuits and intense interests

Despite his anxiety, my goal is to encourage the exploration of his sexuality and attendant worries. The Body Book is a place where we can house and explore any of his ideas. At a point like this in the course of psychotherapy, the therapist functions in part as an affect

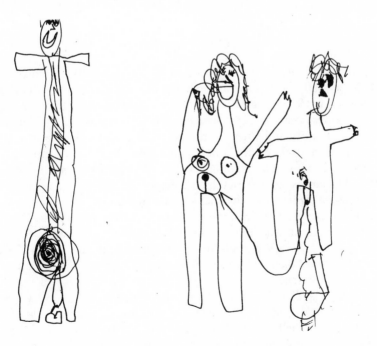

FIGURE 11.2 Andy's Body Book drawings.

regulator. He conveys the idea that although these are intense issues for the child, they can be explored slowly and defused as words and thoughts are added to these affects and play events.

As Andy produced this material, my thoughts went back to some of the diagnostic issues that emerged in the evaluation. Why has Andy not been able to enter the oedipal period? Are we seeing evidence of an excessive amount of castration anxiety? With some children who have many prominent aggressive pre-oedipal conflicts, the "aggressivization" of the punishing father inhibits the emergence of oedipal themes. The child's emotional life remains regressed at an anal level (with Andy the object relation with mother has those features). My goal is to make these phase-appropriate affects less frightening for Andy. The Body Book concretely provides permission to explore these ideas privately.

Although Andy has some explicit sexual conflicts, it is important for the child therapist to explore the child's sexual life in all treatment cases. Sexual issues are a source of tension for children at all stages of development. In the child therapist's role as a developmental facilitator, it is inevitable that sexual questions will arise.

Continuation

In Andy's sessions, he loved to exhibit his growing athletic prowess. He would typically begin a session playing basketball, trying to build up a higher score. He wanted his points to be cumulative—added to the score of a previous hour. He had a strong feeling of pride as the numbers grew larger and larger and I totaled the points and wrote them down.

As he felt excitement about his high score, he would at times tell me new sexual secrets. For example, on one occasion, he whispered conspiratorially that his special friends, the neighborhood boys, have access to *Playboy* magazines. He saw them in the tree house. They are going to give him a copy, and he will sneak it into the house and read it. This "secret" information was followed by telling me about the movie *Fantasia*. This was a very scary movie. There were giants in the movie, and he saw the devil. Andy then announced he is afraid of going to hell. He looked genuinely frightened.

"Holy Mackerel," I note with Andy. "You've become very scared, very frightened, just like you become at home sometimes. You're very worried about hell and that the devil will get you. This worry comes right after you tell me about your strong sexy feelings. I think you have a very mixed-up idea. You think that exciting, sexy feelings are very, very bad, and you make a big punishment for it—in your imagination, the devil will come and get the bad, sexy Andy. *But* everybody who grows up has a lot of strong sexy feelings."

Andy provides many opportunities in this phase of treatment to link punishment fears and lowered self-esteem to the bad sexy impulses he has within him. I clearly indicate that his superego is very harsh, and that sexual thoughts and ideas are found in all boys and girls. This encourages Andy to explore further. In addition, Andy continues to use me on another level as a new object (a developmental facilitator), showing me, with his basketball points, his phallic prowess, that he is feeling enhanced by my encouragement and approval.

Andy works intensely with the Body Book. He studies some of the simple anatomical drawings I made with him showing the differences between men and women. He concentrates on these drawings, and he copies them a number of times. He begins the play of the "naked lady," using the clay we have. He instructs me to make a naked body. I tell him that I will make a general body outline, but he has to make the private parts. He adds the large "boobs" and nipples, a belly button, a rectum, and a "slit" in front with a hole in it. He then makes a large cannonball with spikes in it, which attacks the lady, crushing her arms and legs and then the whole body. This is very intense play, which is repeated over and over again. He has me become the doctor who restores the lady's condition, and then the spiked cannonball returns. I say little about the play, allowing it to evolve.

After playing out this game many times, Andy asks me to build a "naked man." I again construct a figure without genitals. He works hard to fashion a gun out of clay. The man shoots the lady in the "boob," in the rectum, and in the vagina. He wants me to be the screaming lady, saying (with affect) "No . . . No," "Don't," "Help . . . Help," and so forth. He shoots her all over, in the private parts, while she is screaming. The boobs fall off, the nipples fall off, and the arms and legs go as well.

I begin noting with Andy that he is trying to figure out what men and ladies do when they get sexy together. I can see that he has a very strong idea that comes up over and over again—that men hurt ladies when they are excited and sexy. Andy is showing me again his inside ideas. When men and women get naked together, his idea is that the man hurts the woman's private parts. He has a little bit of the right idea—men and ladies touch each other's bodies, but the hurting idea is a mixed-up one. (This kind of comment is made as Andy repeats this intense play, and I also enter some of these ideas in the Body Book with him, through drawings, at the end of the hour.)

Earlier, I discussed the hypothesis that Andy is at the "cusp" of the oedipal period—he evidenced much phallic behavior, but was unable to allow his sexuality to emerge toward his mother. He maintained a regressed, fighting, and controlling (anal) relationship with her. I felt, as the preceding play material unfolded, that we could clearly see the reasons for the developmental impasse. Andy's sexuality was excessively aggressivized. This was due in part to Andy's endowment, parental difficulty in handling his aggression, and the intense rivalry with his sister. Internally, Andy felt that if his sexuality were to emerge, it would be fused with frightening brutality. Therefore, that part of his life had to be denied and ignored. For Andy, it was very dangerous to have a sexy relationship. If left untreated, this would not bode well for Andy's future sexual relationship.

Any work with Andy at this time is aimed at allowing him to feel that he can explore his sexuality. As noted before, the Body Book concretely suggests that he can explore any aspect of his sexual thoughts. He can bring up any intense idea, and we will slowly put these ideas into words, which will defuse some of the raw affect attached to them.

Therefore, as Andy plays out the crushing of the "naked lady," I describe, in words, this powerful unconscious idea he has internally created. He believes that when men get excited with ladies, they hurt them all over. When I verbalize this idea, Andy's rational faculties can be brought into play. He can understand that this is indeed his internal idea—but, in addition, that this idea is a worry that comes from his imagination, and that real sexuality differs from this frightening idea. This insight allows Andy to further explore his sexuality rather than take flight (regress) as we have seen earlier.

For the next few months, in session after session, Andy plays out a variety of themes with the naked lady, in which his oedipal feelings become very evident. He adds the naked man, who has a large penis instead of a gun. He puts the man on top of the woman and says that they should get married together. A number of times, he slips and calls the man "the doctor." He begins to sing "Here comes the bride." Then in the play, he angrily calls out, "*OH YEAH!*" and the figures are attacked and cut into little pieces. I comment directly how boys don't like it when their moms and dads make love. It makes them feel very jealous. Andy tells me to save the pieces of the clay and remake the figures, so we can play the game all over again. This game is repeated again and again. At times, I comment on his word "doctor," noting that I am a grown up man, so Andy feels jealous that I have a wife. Calling out, "OH YEAH!" and initiating an attack on the naked couple is the turning point of each hour. I discuss the fierce "smutch" feelings boys have when they are jealous, feel left out, and feel rejected by the mom.

During several sessions, Andy makes a naked boy, placing him on top of the naked lady. I discuss the strong wishes boys have to do what grown-up daddies do. It's hard to wait all those years until they grow up. Andy responds by putting a mustache on the boy so he can look older and take this special place. Another variation of the play is that after the bride and groom are together, a baby "pops out" of the bride's stomach. He makes the lady with a cavity, a clay baby inside, and he wants the baby to burst out. This allows me to note that he is very curious about how the baby grows and comes out of the mother. I use the Body Book to review conception, pregnancy, and the birth process. I also put a rubber band into the Body Book and discuss how the mommy's small baby hole dilates and expands, allowing the baby to emerge.

Interspersed with the naked lady game, is a new game called "war." We fight each other, and Andy fashions a large, powerful clay gun for himself, whereas I have a small one to use. We shoot at each other, under his direction, and he wounds and kills me. In this game, sometimes he has all the shooters and I have no weapons. As we play, I note that boys really feel bad when they see that their shooter is smaller than their daddy's shooter. They want to have the better shooter. Slowly I can discuss and draw some of the differences between boys and men—the pubic hair, size, how and when sperm is made in addition to urine, and so forth.

Sessions with Parents

During the 6-month period described earlier, the parents reported many gains. They stated that Andy was much more open about his sexual interests. He asked many questions—he wanted clarification as to whether the stork idea (of bringing babies) was true. What did the word "homo" mean? Was it all right to look at ads in magazines of ladies' underwear? The parents were very pleased that Andy could now use words more easily to discuss these difficult topics. They also found a new book, *Where Do I Come From?*, that provided sexual education in a child's format.

Andy was now very affectionate with his mother. He wrote her sweet notes, made special drawings for her, and insisted that she have a day of rest on Mother's Day. He more consistently played harmoniously with his sister, Mary, and was her new guardian in the neighborhood. He also began to develop crushes on girls at school and began skating with a special girl at the roller rink.

Andy began to develop a passion for becoming a pilot. With his parents, he saved money and bought a Topgun leather pilot's jacket, which he loved to wear. He sought special insignias to sew or pin on his jacket and was very excited about photos of himself wearing the jacket. He became interested in books about planes and pilots' lives and involved himself in building fighter models with his father.

Generally, the parents felt that Andy expressed few of his earlier fears. They described him consistently as a youngster who seemed very happy and vibrant and had a good time almost every day. After 6 months of consistent good functioning, Andy was ready for the termination period to begin.

How do we explain what went on in the psychotherapy with Andy in this 6-month period, and why there were significant symptom and behavior changes? In the introduction to this chapter ("The Oedipal Years"), I described the normal oedipal period as one filled with natural conflict. I highlighted that the child becomes anxious about his growing genital sexuality (fears of his sexual affects) and discussed how the new sexuality shapes his object relationships (parents as love objects and rivals). In Andy's case, these conflicts were more difficult to approach because of the problems of aggression unresolved from earlier conflicts. As I discussed before, I felt that the earlier work in treatment made Andy more comfortable and rational about his rivalries, aggression, and "smutch" feelings. With a diminished fear of annihilation and destruction for his rage toward his mother and sister, Andy could allow his sexuality to emerge.

In the treatment hours, Andy began to evidence his strong sexual drive. He was very much interested in nakedness, he was curious about the genitals of men and women, he was trying to understand the process of sexual play and sexual intercourse, and he found it difficult to understand how large babies could emerge from mothers. Andy brought forth these ideas in play action form, and I helped him to put words to the affective ideas. "Dick," "boobs," "vagina," "nipples," " tushi," and "making love" slowly gave us a working vocabulary that we could use together. Thus, I could later discuss with him the differences between "daddies' dicks" and "children's dicks."

In general, these sessions brought secondary process thinking to primary process affects. As we used these ideas, discussed them, and drew or wrote them in the Body Book, much of the frightening affective components became defused. These ideas could be thought about, and this process fostered the neutralization of the drive components.

An accompanying theme that enhanced this kind of exploration, with which I dealt, was Andy's harsh superego reactions. When Andy, for example, confessed about sexual secrets and then feared the devil, I made explicit Andy's thought process. Andy felt that only bad boys thought about sex. The fact that I encouraged such thinking (joined by the parents through the parent work) allowed Andy to begin to modify his superego reactions. Thus, these forbidden feelings could become more conscious, be expressed openly, understood empathically, and become acceptable to Andy himself.

When these forbidden feelings became more acceptable internally, Andy could use these affects in his daily life. He became openly curious about sexual matters with his parents, he could let himself feel his sexuality toward his mother, and he could develop crushes on girls. Thus, the repressed sexual affects became available and used in his daily life in a phase-appropriate way. During the latency period to follow, many of these feelings will again be repressed, but the fact that they were available during the oedipal years lays the foundation for a healthy sexuality for Andy in the future.

During the course of the "naked lady" play, Andy expressed many typical oedipal conflicts. One theme involved his smallness in comparison to grown-up men. No matter how many points he built up, or how big a shooter he erected from clay, grown-up men (his father and his doctor) had special equipment he did not have. This is a typical form of narcissistic injury that oedipal children need to acknowledge and slowly accept. Another narcissistic "blow" was that the naked lady would only choose the naked man to sleep with. He could destroy the marital couple again and again, he could kill the bride's groom, but slowly he had to accept the sexual rejection. In his play, we see that Andy began to take steps in the coping process. He found his own girlfriend at the skating rink. Thus, we see signs of displacement of his sexual feelings from mother to peers. He worked with his father on his pilot interest. While he felt like a grown-up man wearing his pilot jacket (a typical form of denial), he began to read about pilots and build models. Thus, we began to see the early process of sublimation, a delay of immediate gratification, which enhances the process of coping with the oedipal drives.

As we worked together, it was helpful to the treatment process to follow several components of my relationship with Andy. One component was the transference. *Andy developed a father transference within the sessions. His "doctor" slip equated father and therapist, who lay on top of the naked lady. He developed "war" with me, and by turning passive into active, he had the larger gun. I became synonymous with father. In the treatment hour, Andy was jealous that I had a wife and rageful that I had more potent equipment. Therefore, when I could describe these affects that he was experiencing toward me (as well as his father) at the moment, he could resonate to my understanding. He experienced relief when I discussed the normative context for his feelings—for example, how all boys feel very angry when they feel smaller.*

Despite the intensity of negative feelings toward me in the transference, Andy's bond with me grew in this period. Mr. Chethik became a special man who understood his play, who put his scary play into words, and who then helped him take away anxiety and bad self-feelings. This bond stemmed from the growing therapeutic alliance (another component of the relationship). The treatment setting became a special place where Andy allowed frightening internal events to emerge and experienced relief.

After a year of work together, I evaluated the process. For a sustained period of time, Andy was not symptomatic in his outer functioning. He was not self-attacking or abusive. Rivalry toward Mary had markedly diminished, and his relationship with his mother had become positive (including periods of sexualization). He generally was functioning well in school and with peers, and there was a sense of pleasure, playfulness, and vibrancy in his life. I felt that Andy had internally dealt with significant aspects of phase-appropriate oedipal conflicts, and I could see some beginning steps toward latency. Therefore, I could support the parents' wish now to begin termination.

Termination

The termination period should be conceived as a discrete phase with a beginning, a middle, and an end. It should commence after an assessment, which is used as a base. In child therapy the rational reasons should first be discussed with the parents, and then with the child. It is important that the termination period be long enough to deal with some of the feelings of loss and separation that inevitably are evoked. It is also helpful to establish a clear, specific date that establishes clearly the reality of the ending.

After a discussion and agreement with his parents, I talked directly with Andy. I described some of the worries he had when he began—he thought he was the worst boy in the world, he was scared of ghosts and the dark, and he was also very angry with his mom and Mary. I felt that through our play and thinking in the office, and with the help of his mom and dad at home, we came to know about his inside feelings and worries. I felt he was no longer upset about his inside feelings, and this helped him to be happy now and feel good about himself. Because we were finishing our work together, I suggested that we should take some time to say good-bye and then stop our work.

Andy, at first, showed no direct response to these ideas, but his play changed. He began to play basketball by himself, no longer wanting me to participate or keep score. I commented that he was throwing me out of the game and that I thought he was doing this because he felt thrown out by me. For several sessions, when Andy uncharacteristically went into some form of solitary play (e.g., basketball, or drawing with his back to me), I suggested that he was making believe I wasn't there. He felt I didn't care about him—he was angry and hurt, so he was getting even by turning his back on me. I really wasn't throwing him out at all—we were really close to finishing our work. This was like the end of the year with his teacher. He no longer went to his old class, and he would no longer see his teacher. He would miss his teacher—not because he was thrown out, but because he was promoted. With these comments, Andy moved in and out of interaction with me.

Andy and I constructed a calendar together, and we counted the number of meetings we would have left (eight sessions, a 2-month period). I noted that he had a full private drawer of books, papers, drawings, and clay creations to go through, and that he and I had to decide what he would do with these contents. Andy's initial response was to bring up the wastepaper basket and proceed to dump everything into it. I stopped that process, returned the contents to the drawer, and suggested that Andy was showing me that he still felt those angry thrown-out feelings, so he was trashing everything we did together. (Actually, Andy now openly expressed his anger and hurt at home, telling his parents that he didn't want to come anymore and breaking into tears, saying that I didn't like him. His parents had an opportunity to listen to his intense feelings and to explain to him why we were taking these steps.)

In the last five sessions, Andy worked more freely, slowly deciding who would keep the things we created together. He definitely wanted to keep his excellent drawings and take them home; he felt I should keep his Body Book because that was "private," but he wanted the "Smutch Book" for himself. Clay objects and houses made of Legos were taken apart and returned to the common toy area where they could be used by others. Andy wanted to know whether I would keep one of his pictures on the wall, and he also brought in several of his recent snapshots—hitting a baseball and wearing his Topgun leather jacket. I told him that I couldn't keep his picture on the wall, but maybe he was a little worried that I might forget him. I told Andy that he would definitely "stick in my mind."

We ended by planning a special party for the last session. Andy brought the drinks, and my assignment was to supply the Twinkies. I talked about how I would miss him and that I knew his mom and dad planned to let me know how he was doing. Andy sought to hide his sad feelings by pulling down the brim of his baseball cap.

In the termination period, one should anticipate that ambivalence will emerge. On one hand, patients often feel enhanced by a sense of approval and accomplishment. But this process also stimulates old responses to perceived loss and rejection. Andy turned his back on me (turning passive into active) because he felt that I was abandoning him. I felt that part of Andy's response was to re-experience the earlier sibling rejection he perceived. I was forgetting him and would give my attention to a new needy child—a repetition, in his feelings, of Mary's arrival in the family. Although I described some of his responses in the treatment hour, the major affects of loss, rage, and sadness were actually experienced and verbalized at home with his parents.

In this ending phase, the concretization process continues to be utilized and has a special role with the child patient. Specifically, we made a calendar together. Andy marked off each session with an "X," measuring the time we had left. As our sessions dwindled down, we tangibly divided up and emptied the contents of Andy's private drawer. This process brings home to children the reality of separation and ending because it is done through concrete action.

Addendum: Denial of Childhood Sexuality

The case of Andy provides an opportunity to discuss some current issues of childhood sexuality that permeate our culture and national consciousness. I have been struck that when I present the preceding clinical material, as a teacher or colleague with professional groups, people raise the following questions. "What happened to Andy?" "What kind of sexual events did he experience?" "Was he sexually abused?" The implication is that a youngster with this kind of sexual fantasy life must have suffered traumatic reality experiences. These common reactions reflect a significant lack of understanding about childhood sexual development. They are symbolic of the national hyperawareness of sexual abuse, supported by large segments of the mental health community.

A major problem in our diagnostic and assessment processes is that many child "experts" do not understand the intensity of the growing child's natural sexual life and fantasy preoccupations. All young children, who see the world from a body-egocentric point of view, attempt to sort out all kinds of issues about sexuality. They are intensely involved in sexual research: What are the differences between boys and girls? Do girls lose their "wieners," and were they boys once? Can I also lose my wiener? How are babies made? Does the stork bring them? Do doctors make the babies in the hospital? How do babies get inside? Do babies grow because mommies eat a lot? Why do mommies and daddies sleep together? Do they get naked together? Does daddy put something into mommy's tushi? How does the baby come out? Is there an explosion when the baby comes out? Does the baby come out of the tushi?

As we work in psychotherapy with children, these attempts to understand and sort out reality will naturally emerge. On the way to putting together a relatively real concept of the body, love, conception, and birth, all sorts of hypotheses are developed and discarded. Oral concepts (pregnancy through eating), anal concepts (e.g., birth by defecation), phallic concepts (e.g., swords, stabbing the lady) are typical expressions of these intense preoccupations, and they are specifically shaped by the individual child's sensitivities. Because Andy struggled with pre-oedipal aggressive conflicts, his sexual fantasies were "aggressivized" as he sought to understand the world.

This natural body of sexual preoccupation is often misunderstood by child therapists and seen as "evidence" of sexual abuse or some form of real sexual overstimulation. In fact, the last 10 to 15 years has seen the birth of a specialized cottage industry of sexual abuse experts, armed with anatomical dolls, who claim to be able to ferret out the truth when sexual abuse is alleged. It has been my experience that many of these experts tap into the natural sexual fantasies of childhood in their clinical interviews, and this is often the basis for their evidence of abuse. Implicitly, many practitioners deny that all children are unconsciously dealing with the sexual world.

There is little doubt that sexual abuse does occur, and it has enormous impact on a child's development. However, it is always accompanied with significant evidence of regression and nonfunctioning in many areas of a child's life. While Andy uncovered violent forms of sexual intercourse in his play, he functioned very effectively at school, at home, and within the community. A traumatized child is one whose ego is overwhelmed. Typically dramatic and far-reaching changes are evident in the child's daily life when sexual abuse occurs: sleep disruption, significant withdrawal, clinging to safe objects, general deterioration of ego functioning. Even with these changes, one must be cautious about confirming sexual abuse, inasmuch as the added findings would suggest only that they are consistent with the *possibility* of sexual trauma. Other traumas (e.g., significant separation, surgery, etc.) can also cause these reactions in childhood.

I feel it is imperative that child therapists understand the natural sexual issues that all children struggle to comprehend as they develop.

BIBLIOGRAPHY

Freud, S. (1905). *Three Essays on Sexuality* (Standard Ed., Vol. 13). London: Hogarth Press.

Freud, S. (1908). *On the Sexual Theories of Children* (Standard Ed., Vol. 9). Longdon: Hogarth Press.

Freud, S. (1924). *Dissolution of the Oedipus Complex* (Standard Ed., Vol. 19). London: Hogarth Press.

Nagera, H. (1966). Early childhood disturbances, neurosis and the adult disturbances. *Psychoanalytic Study of the Child*. New York: International University Press.

Nagera, H. (1991). The four-to-six stage. In: S. Greenspan & G. Pollack (eds.), *The Course of Life*, Vol. III, *Middle to Late Childhood*. Conn: International University Press.

Nagera, H. (1996). Early childhood disturbances, neurosis, and the adult disturbances. *Psychoanalytic Study of the Child*. New York: International University Press.

VanDorn, H. (1991). The Oedipus complex revisited. In: S. Greenspan & G. Pollack (Eds.), *The Course of Life*, Vol. III, *Middle to Late Childhood*. Conn: International University Press.

12

~

The Case of Margaret M

INTRODUCTION: THE LATENCY YEARS

The material in this chapter will focus on the evaluation and treatment of a 7-year-old girl. As in the first case in Part IV, the diagnostic process will be initially presented, followed by the unfolding psychotherapy with the child, as well as the parent work throughout the course of the treatment.

Our considerations about this little girl in early latency must be placed in a developmental context. What normative and pathogenic considerations would we have in mind concerning latency as we assess the specific material of a 7-year-old?

In his discussion of childhood sexuality, Freud (1905) noted that the child's sexual life is "diphasic"—it grows in early childhood, culminating in the oedipal period; it is interrupted during the latency years; and it reemerges in early adolescence, spurred by the further development of the pubertal drive. The developmental "interruption" is fostered by two major internal factors that converge simultaneously: One is psychological, promoted by the dissolution of the oedipal conflict; the second is maturational, promoted by ego development (the thinking, perceiving, rational parts of the child).

In the introduction to the previous case, we began discussing how the oedipal child gradually moves away from overt sexual longing and rivalry related to his parents because of both castration anxiety (imagined threat) and repeated narcissistic disappointments and injury (the parent union remains a formidable reality). The sexual and aggressive drives are repressed; they now become dormant and "latent" because, as noted earlier, their emergence will produce both intense anxiety and ongoing frustration. In addition, the young child now has resources that empower her ego, which helps her to build a defensive barrier to the unconscious and to find alternative pleasures. The normal maturation of her mind and thinking processes, particularly the shift to concrete operational thinking (see Piaget, 1967; Shapiro, 1976), enhances her ability to learn and understand the real world around her. In normal development, the ego becomes enhanced during these years, shifting some power from the id. During this "age of reason," a new form of pleasure (sublimation) becomes available as the child solves problems, learns, and uses her growing ability to understand and participate in the outside world. This occurs in school as well as in less formal settings.

There are a number of considerations to follow as we evaluate the progress of latency:

1. *Struggle with masturbation.* Although the drives are repressed, there continues to be much internal pressure for their expression, and the child fears breakthroughs of these feelings in the form of masturbation. We often see children establish compulsive rituals and obsessions at this age so as to remain "in control." Sleep problems tend to emerge, because the drives are often stronger in the quiescent period before sleep. Many young latency-age children also displace their physical sexual feelings into whole-body discharge; this is a period in which wrestling, gymnastics, soccer, and other general physical activity are on the ascendence.

2. *Superego development.* Freud (1924) noted that the "heir of the oedipal period is the superego." During the earlier years, the child slowly takes in the prohibitions and sanctions of her parents, but with a powerful need to effectively repress the forbidden drives of childhood in latency, the sanctioning part of the mind (the superego) becomes consolidated and much more effective as an internal controlling institution. Controls (set off by feelings of shame and guilt) are now less dependent on the adults around the child and emerge more often from the standards and values within the child's mind. Thus, we note that self-esteem regulation is now predominantly controlled from within—for example, the child feels internally enhanced because she has done a good job on her homework, or she

feels "down" because she has not finished it—even when the teacher has not seen her work.

3. *Object relations*. With some dissolution of the intense libidinal ties within the home, there is a shift toward new adult authority (and new identifications) and peers outside the home. Teachers quickly become a new authority, and one often hears the early-latency child intone, "But my teacher says. . . ." Peers and friendships become increasingly important and replace some of the libidinal attachments toward the family. The process of socialization to the outside world is enhanced by how the child manages with her latency friends, and further separation achievements occur through sleep-overs and summer overnight camp, particularly likely in this period.

4. *Fantasy and play*. Because of the development of the mind (ego's growth), the child becomes able to use thinking rather than direct action. She can express and experience earlier pleasures through her fantasy life, which grows extensively. Now, for example, rather than having a need for guns and swords used directly in play, a young boy becomes very invested in comic books or *Star Trek* and becomes extensively involved in following the episodes and the development of a character. He now lives out his "power" in thought and imagination as a "Trekkie" rather than directly shooting and stabbing with his play guns and swords. A young girl collects pictures of rock stars from magazines, rather than live out the crushes within her family or play school.

The play of latency youngsters characteristically also turns to games with other peers. Play at this age enhances the socialization process. Competition, expression of the aggressive drive, continues, but this expression has to fit into the new society surrounding the child. In latency groups, there is typically endless discussion of the rules, the scoring process, fairness and cheating. While the child is developing skills and abilities, she must fit into the group standards and mores. This is an important foundation for living in the larger society in the future.

5. *Sublimation*. Another important index of latency is the child's ability to sublimate the more primitive instinctual drives. Does she begin to get pleasure from her creative activities and achievements, and is there some neutralization of the drives? In the course of development, direct instinctual expression is typically not sanctioned by parents, outside authorities, or the growing internal

superego. Can the developing youngster find alternate, deflected means for expression? The ego growth of latency provides a rich opportunity. For example, some youngsters in latency become avid writers or artists-in-the-making, using these new ego skills. These creations can contain important gratifying themes, but they are expressed in forms that are acceptable by the surrounding authorities. Gradually, these activities become a fundamental source of pleasure themselves. Although I have highlighted artistic pleasure, these changes may be expressed in a variety of ego activities such as the development of sports and body skills.

As we assess the 7-year-old youngster, we initially need to ask whether she has been able to reach the latency phase of development. Is she still struggling with oedipal issues too intensively, and are there legacies of the oral and anal periods that are unresolved?

In addition, how is she struggling with the previously defined developmental considerations of latency? What is the quality of her superego functioning—is it too permissive, allowing many breakthroughs, or unduly harsh and punitive? Is she separating effectively from the primary members of her family and able to make friends and play easily with peers? How do her teachers react to her? Does she appear to be developing her skills and abilities to learn effectively, and do these achievements provide a source of pleasure for her?

The Evaluation of Margaret M and Her Family

Margaret was almost 7 years old at the time of the evaluation. She came from an intact, upper-middle-class family; her father was an executive in a small company, and her mother was a teacher in a public school system. Both parents were in their early 30s. Their youngest child, Seth, was 7 months old.

Presenting Problems

Both parents were available for the three appointments to discuss the presenting problems of Margaret, her developmental history, and their own history, courtship, and marriage. The mother was more of a driving force behind the evaluation, though the father "agreed" with the concerns expressed.

Generally, her mother felt that Margaret was an extremely bossy and controlling young lady. She constantly ordered her friends around, had to decide what they played, and often talked to the teacher about the "misbehavior" of some of her classmates. She seemed to continue to have friends because she had many leadership qualities, but all occasions with peers were marked with fighting and demands.

Margaret seemed very angry with her mother much of the time. She complained about all of her mother's normal daily demands, and she dawdled and resisted. There had been a constant struggle with her mother about food and eating for many years. For example, Margaret hated meat loaf, wouldn't touch a "charred" hotdog, and had a long list of food avoidances. Lunch could consist of only a few foods and had to be packaged in a special ways—all items folded neatly in plastic in the lunch box.

Margaret's complaints also extended to school. A major theme was that "things aren't fair." A classmate had more time to do her work; someone touched her desk and moved her things; kids were mean. She complained that these distractions kept her from getting the best grades in tests and papers, although, in reality, she did extremely well.

The parents also discussed other forms of growing perfectionism. It could take Margaret a very long time to pick out just the right thing to wear, and at least 20 minutes to fold her socks in just the right way. She would practice her ballet steps till she did them perfectly, and she would become obsessed with practicing until she reached that goal. In recent months her perfectionism was expanding and absorbing more energy. Although Margaret could perform well in many areas, she had little pleasure in her achievements because she was preoccupied with not making a mistake.

In the past year Margaret has also been experiencing bad dreams, which disturbed her sleep; she reacted with tension to the anticipation of going to bed and continued to battle with her parents to delay her bedtime.

I was concerned about how the parents presented this initial material about Margaret. The mother's speech was very pressured, which evidenced a great deal of anxiety about her daughter. I wondered what could be causing this quality of anxiety. The father did not join as fully in describing the daughter's problems. Did he agree with the mother's assessment? When I noticed his reticence, I asked at several points, "Do you see things the same way?" Although he nominally agreed, was he being compliant or assuaging some intense need of the mother, rather than sharing his own real opinion?

It is not unusal to pick up important differences between parents in their assessment of their child or their motivation for treatment for the child. Because treatment is a major family undertaking, it is important to flesh out these differences early so that the treatment will not be undercut midway. Ideally, this should be done during the evaluation or feedback session. These differences in the parents produced an internal uneasiness within me and alerted me to the need to understand more about the parental motivation for this treatment.

Developmental History

Margaret's history has to be seen in the light of a troubled marriage during the child's earliest years. The parents had been married for a total of 10 years at the time of the evaluation. Mrs. M became pregnant with Margaret when they were married for about 2 years, and Mr. M returned to graduate school for an advanced degree in business. He began having an affair during the pregnancy, and although the mother was aware that "something was wrong," the affair came to light only when Margaret was 30 months old. A separation followed; Margaret saw her father on Wednesdays and weekends for 1 year. The parents began dating each other and reunited a year after the separation began. The father moved back into the home when Margaret was 4 years old. Shortly after, the mother became pregnant, and Seth was born when Margaret was more than 6 years old.

The mother has always felt that there has been a strain in her relationship with Margaret. There was never a problem with Margaret's development or achievements. Her walking and talking milestones were all achieved early, and Margaret was considered a bright and capable child by her preschool teachers. The strain her mother felt was in relation to Margaret's moods. During the first year of life, Margaret cried a good deal. Her mother felt she was not enjoying her baby; she was jealous of her friends who seemed to be at greater ease with their children. This tension has been ongoing. Mrs. M recalled that her "life would be on hold until the baby would take her nap." She now felt a great deal of guilt, as she was aware that she could be really comfortable with Seth, the second child. She recalled not letting Margaret cry as a baby, because she felt it reflected badly on her as a mother. She was eager to go back to work and did so when Margaret was 6 months old (half-time as a teacher).

Mrs. M felt that there was a constant struggle with Margaret during her toddler years. There were struggles over food, and Margaret became a very picky eater. In addition, she would always make her mother wait if there were somewhere to go, as well as make demands that she knew her mother could not fulfill at the moment. It seemed as if there were a constant control battle. Toilet training was absolutely no problem, because it was clear that Margaret wanted to be trained. But if there was anything Margaret did not want to do, which was a daily occurrence, the battle would ensue. The mother said that she could get very angry—she never spanked Margaret but became a "screamer and yeller." (Her mother discussed this with a lot of apparent anxiety and guilt, often comparing these negative reactions to the positive feelings she had with Seth.)

Simultaneously, she knew there were problems in her marriage—there were long stretches when the couple had no sex— and both parents retrospectively felt that this marital tension affected Mrs. M's parenting. When the affair finally came to light, there was an intense blowup between the parents, and the mother actually experienced a great deal of relief after the blowup. The father and mother separated immediately on mother's demand, and father curtailed the extramarital relationship at that time. The mother pursued the separation (the father was against it), and during the course of the separation the mother dated and felt her experience of being wanted by others helped to restore her self-esteem. But the mother always felt that she loved her husband and responded positively when he began courting her again. The father said he knew he had made a terrible mistake, and from the start of the separation worked for their reunion.

Currently, there is some division between the parents about Margaret. Her father agreed that Margaret could be very nasty; he felt she did not get along with her mother and was aware of his daughter's mood difficulties and symptoms. But he felt he could work with her, calm her down, and reason with her. He thought that, when handled calmly, Margaret was quite malleable. It was her mother's approach that was too confrontational.

Her father also felt that Margaret was wonderful. She was a great dancer and often performed for him. She did a wonderful impersonation of Katarina Witt, the figure skater. They also did many things together on weekends—shopping and gardening. Margaret was very affectionate with her father.

Mrs. M felt that she was often angry with Margaret. If her father cooked breakfast and made pancakes, Margaret would eat very well, but her mother's pancakes were inedible. The mother remarked that there was a marked division in the house: father and daughter on one side, and mother and son on the other.

This material began to give me an understanding of the different emotional attitudes the parents exhibited about Margaret.

Some of the mother's anxiety and pressured speech seemed to be driven by her intense guilt about the long-standing negative feelings she carried for her daughter. She appeared very anxious about what she was exposing about herself, and I suspected she was fearful that she had significantly impaired her daughter's development.

I felt I understood why the father seemed to be temporizing about Margaret. It appeared he was aware of Margaret's difficulties (moodiness, problems with peers and mother), but he seemed to be expressing a need to protect his daughter. Was he implying that Margaret would be fine if her mother was calmer with her and handled their daughter as he did? Did he temporize because of guilt about the affair?

I felt at this point that there were indeed major divisions in attitudes toward Margaret. I wondered whether some of these attitudes might in some way be connected to the marital discord that disrupted the marriage during Margaret's early years.

Parents' Background

Mr. M is the youngest of three brothers from an upper-middle-class family. His father was also a businessman, but not considered successful. He was characterized as an introvert and generally ineffective. Mr. M felt that he came from a "strong matriarchal family." His mother was the dominant force, and she was always "closer to her three sons than the father was." The mother and sons formed a strong unit within the family; the father was an outsider. The mother was a charismatic person in the community. She had strong political views and was elected to several local political positions.

Both of Margaret's parents felt uneasy with the past relationship that Mr. M's mother attempted to foster with her three sons. It was clear that this grandmother felt that her son's marriage and decision to live in a distant community were a sign of disloyalty to her. Mr.

M's brothers have remained in the original family orbit, but the grandmother has cut off contact with the "disloyal son."

Margaret's mother was the younger of two daughters. Her father was a very successful businessman who was out of the country, on business, for long periods of time. Everyone in the family was terrified of the father, who had a reputation for being "tyrannical." Mrs. M felt her mother never developed her capabilities but gave herself up for her husband and children. Mrs. M has always feared that these "martyr-like qualities" might filter down to her. She recalls playing the guitar for several years, but giving it up because her father announced that he hated that instrument. The tension in Mrs. M's orginal home was ever present.

Interviews with Margaret

Margaret was a very pretty, quite thin, meticulous-looking 7-year-old. She was attractively dressed, and her long blonde, braided hair was striking.

Margaret initially surveyed my office, looked out the window, and said, "It would be a test if I had to jump out." (My office is on the 19th floor.) I commented that she might be very scared of coming to see me.

When I asked what her parents told her about coming, she told me that she talks with her dad alot. She has worries at night, when she goes to sleep and is separated from her parents. She thinks about biting vampires. Last night she dreamed that a girl was walking into the mouth of a giant vampire.

She began to use the art supplies in the room; a picture story emerged of a princess with long, braided hair, who who was walking in the woods carrying a basket. She drew a castle in the background. In the story the princess found a little bunny. She brought the bunny back to the castle and asked her mother whether she could keep it. Her mother gave her permission, and she was happy to keep her pet. The drawing was creative; Margaret had a good deal of skill and used multiple media simultaneously. The long golden hair of the princess was made from clay, so that it had a three-dimensional quality as it lay on the paper.

In the second session, Margaret again quickly became absorbed in her multiple-media project. Another forest scene developed in which the princess was walking. On one of the branches of a tree was a dangerous snake (made out of clay). The snake had a bad disease and was infecting everything in the forest. Margaret expressed this idea in the picture by taking bits of gray clay and "infecting" tree branches, trunks, and so on. The disease spread everywhere, and even the princess finally became infected. When this occurred, Margaret shuddered. She was greatly absorbed in this project, which we put into her private drawer to be worked on in the future.

During both sessions I talked about the worries Margaret clearly had. I noted that she was upset about going to sleep and about her frightening dreams, like the one about the vampire. I could even see how scared she became as she worked on the drawings. Inside feelings, I said, were upsetting her. Because she can express her imagination freely, this may help us find out what her inside worries are about.

Psychodynamic Technical Assessment

The purpose of our assessment is to define the problem areas and to understand what factors are creating the difficulties. Margaret's problems fall into several areas: anxieties and symptoms, character issues, and external problems.

Margaret's need to be perfect appeared to be a growing symptom. Her need to perform without making a mistake was consuming an increased amount of her energy and appeared to impede her work and play. Anxiety also appeared to be breaking through at night, expressed in her dreams.

Margaret was developing extensive bossy and controlling qualities—character issues—which were permeating many relationships. She expressed anger and a need for dominance in these interactions.

Margaret's need to battle with her mother was not only driven by her internal feelings, but was often stimulated by external issues. Her mother was angry often, and Margaret reacted to this external provocation.

I. Drive Assessment

Despite the fact that Margaret is a latency-aged girl, she is in the midst of a severe, ongoing oedipal conflict. She appears to be in an intense family triangulation—sexual wishes for her father and rivalry with her mother. In her evaluation session, through her art work and attendant stories she lives out her wish for a baby (the princess finds the bunny/baby and receives the queen's permission to keep it). Her sexual interest becomes frightening, expressed when the snake/penis spreads a fearsome disease. The oedipal themes are not only lived out in fantasy, but expressed in daily living. Father is "close" to his daughter and mother is often is the rival who is left out.

This stage fixation is problematic for a latency-aged youngster. In addition, there is evidence of pre-oedipal drive struggles. Oral and anal themes emerge in Margaret's relationship with her mother. The oral struggles are suggested through Margaret's fights with mother over food and her worries about being devoured by vampires. Anal themes are expressed in the withholding and ongoing passive–aggressive struggles with her mother.

II. Ego Assessment

Margaret is a very well-endowed youngster, and her ego functions are highly developed. She is bright and creative, as evidenced in her superior school functioning and her art projects.

As noted earlier, Margaret has internal conflicts on a number of levels. She appears to have a great deal of guilt about her oedipal wishes (both sexual and rivalrous) and seeks punishment through her frightening dream activity. The defense of *projection* is utilized—her self-attack is projected to frightening figures in her dreams (e.g., vampires) that are out to get her. Earlier aggressive conflicts with her mother are expressed behaviorally. She fights her mother through food, rejecting her mother's nurturing offers, and through her passive–aggressive behaviors. In addition, she wards off some of her mother's attack by the mechanism of *identification with the aggressor*, which Margaret uses extensively. Rather than submitting to her mother's criticalness, Margaret herself becomes the angry attacker, particularly with peers.

Margaret struggles extensively with her mother's displeasure with her, which has been lifelong. The material suggests that the mother's rejection creates significant narcissistic injury within Margaret. She internally experiences depression and loss of self-esteem, but she appears to defend vigorously against these affects by her driven *perfectionism*. This is her attempt to retain a "superior" feeling about herself, pushing away any depressed images.

III. Superego Assessment

Margaret has a fully developed internalized superego that seems to be working overtime and making her life difficult. Her superego appears to be both harsh and demanding. Two sources that fuel her strong conscience are her early aggression turned inward and her perception of her mother's lifelong discomfort with her.

The oedipal sexual drives and aggressive rivalry toward her

mother (both oedipal and preoedipal) are forbidden and produce guilt initially and a need for punishment secondarily. The most prominent manifestation of this guilt/punishment dynamic is the nightly bad dreams. The "bad girl" during the day finds a way to hurt herself during the night by experiencing terror at the hands of a monster/vampire.

As noted earlier, the mother's discomfort with her daughter has been incorporated by Margaret, and she often feels "there is something wrong with me." She experiences a loss of self-esteem as well as an accompanying depression. She vigorously fights these unpleasurable states, using a number of defenses. As she *identifies with the aggressor*, the attacking, belittling Margaret proclaims that she is not defective, but that the others surrounding her are indeed the defectives ones. Similarly, she uses *perfectionism* to quiet her internal attacks. It is as if she is saying that if she constantly performs perfectly, no disabling self-demeaning feelings will ever reach her. Because her internal attack is persistent, her need for perfectionism spreads.

IV. Genetic–Dynamic Formulation

The parents' marriage was strained during Margaret's early years. This appeared to have had a significant impact on the mother's relationship with her daughter. The mother was always uneasy and uncomfortable with her. This underlying state produced early difficulties in her caring for her daughter. Margaret appears to have reacted early, as expressed by battles in regard to food and feeding and the daily battles about compliance to her mother's requests and expectations.

The angry struggle with mother was carried into the oedipal period, making competitive rivalry with the mother more intense. The evaluation revealed that Margaret remained locked in an unresolved oedipal struggle.

This internal struggle was exacerbated by the parents' handling of Margaret. Her father functioned as the good, caring, closely attuned parent, therefore solidifying a loving, oedipal tie. Her mother continued to be the estranged, impatient, critical, "yeller and screamer," further solidfying the anger in Margaret.

Margaret should be further along in her latency development. Much of her energy is bound up in her relationships with her parents. During latency, a shift in her attachment to her outside objects should begin. The inflamed nature of Margaret's current conflicts makes this shift very difficult.

Because of Margaret's basic ego ability, she performs at a very high level. Does her performance meet the latency criteria for effective sublimination? Does her ability to achieve serve her as a new source of pleasure? Unfortunately, Margaret gets very little pleasure from her achievements, and they are used primarily to quell anxious doubts that continuously bubble up within her.

V. Treatment Recommendations

I recommended twice-weekly, insight-oriented psychotherapy for Margaret. Like Andy, she evidenced many strengths that would make her a good candidate for uncovering treatment. Her ego functions were intact and, indeed, well developed. She used her imagination well and could play out her ideas skillfully, and she had the ability to connect with her therapist. In addition, in contrast to Andy, as an older latency youngster, Margaret had a better capacity for self-reflection. During the evaluation, when I pointed out how she suffered from bad dreams, Margaret seemed to understand the need for a "worry doctor."

Weekly sessions were recommended for the parents. The work with the parents in this case seemed to be very important. A major goal would be to help the mother understand her relationship with Margaret and to develop a capacity for empathy with her daughter. Another important goal with the parents was to shift some of the current balances in the family. The "good father/bad mother" split seemed to be the most immediate dynamic to address, and this constellation inflamed Margaret's oedipal turmoil. The thrust of my work with the parents would encompass the techniques of parent guidance, as well as "treatment of the parent–child relationship" (see Chapters 4 and 5).

Feedback Interview. Margaret and her parents all came to the feedback session, but I divided the hour so that I could meet with the parents separately from Margaret.

Initially, I saw the parents without Margaret. I indicated that during the evaluation I felt they expressed differences about Margaret's need for treatment. The mother seemed eager, whereas the father was more questioning. I told the parents that as I presented my ideas about Margaret, I felt it was very important that they both feel free to react honestly and fully.

I said that Margaret impressed me as an intelligent and gifted young girl, but she was developing some problems. I agreed with the impression that she was becoming disdainful, abrasive and demeaning of others. This pattern seemed to be growing (a character problem) and could become entrenched and permanent. I felt Margaret used this to make herself feel better; she was the "criticizer" rather than the one being criticized.

I also explained that her "perfectionism" served a similar purpose. Being absolutely excellent was her attempt to push away an inside worry that she was flawed. For Margaret, it was an endless battle—whatever she did was never good enough and couldn't silence her internal doubt.

My task in my work with Margaret would be to help her become more aware of these negative inside self-perceptions and to see how inaccurate they were.

I also outlined the need for weekly sessions with the parents—to work on undoing the "good parent/bad parent" split and to help the mother understand the tension between herself and her daughter.

The father was much more forthcoming than I had anticipated, and I felt this occurred because of my introductory remarks. He agreed with my ideas about his daughter and her need for some therapy. He also felt that there were very real problems between his wife and himself in their perception of Margaret. He intuitively did not like the split that had developed, but somehow had felt "forced" to take the role he had. He felt his wife was impatient, angry with their daughter, and always on her case. He tried to show his wife that it wasn't so difficult to get along with Margaret and that she responded to understanding. He felt he took Margaret's side because she often seemed so bereft after a fight with her mother. Yet he knew the way things were currently handled was a real mess. He was glad that I would work with them, because they needed some help.

The mother agreed that they indeed had a lot of work to do. She said that Margaret's father couldn't understand that no matter what she did, her daughter reacted differently to her than she did to her father. She was glad that the father finally said openly what was on his mind.

During the latter part of the session I saw Margaret alone.

Margaret showed no overt response to my informing her that we will continue to meet together to work out her worries. She registered a lot of pleasure in finding that she now had a private drawer and that her special creations were placed there safely.

Treatment Implications

As we began therapy, how would we anticipate and define the *treatment goals*, and what kinds of *resistances* and *transferences* could potentially emerge?

Treatment Goals

Many of Margaret's drives are repressed and defended from consciousness. Her rage and competitiveness toward her mother and her sexualized feelings toward her father were forbidden, and a goal would be to help Margaret become aware of these feelings and to accept such affects as part of growing up. This potential awareness would reduce her underlying guilt.

Similarly, it would be very important to help her understand her drivenness, expressed in her need to be perfect. Needing to be the best allowed Margaret to push away the strong worries she had about herself. Her need to put down other people also kept away the worry that other people would attack her. An important goal would be to help her become aware that she had strong self-doubts and to help her understand why they had developed.

Achieving these goals with Margaret was predicated on helping to make some shifts within the mother and between the parents.

Resistances

We can certainly anticipate that Margaret will have an enormously difficult time allowing herself to feel momentarily small, frightened, helpless and defective. These are the affects she experienced as a young child in her relationship with her mother. Margaret has understandably gone to great lengths to ward off any depression, and in many ways her active coping must be seen as a strength. In therapy she will have an opportunity to face her self-doubts without being overwhelmed by them.

Transference

Margaret, we can predict, will express many of her father/oedipal attachments in her relationship with the therapist. I anticipate that I will become an exciting object whom she will want to win. This transference will give me opportunities to talk about her "special daddy feelings," aspects of which make her feel very guilty.

There is also a possibility that further along in the treatment, Margaret will experience me as the depriving mother. This kind of reemerging object tie can potentially give us entry into Margaret's early years with her mother.

THE FIRST MONTH OF TREATMENT SESSIONS WITH MARGARET

In this period I want to focus more clearly on the details of a treatment hour, and I will be using Margaret's first sessions after the evaluation to highlight the treatment process. I also want to describe how I gradually set up the atmosphere for treatment.

Early in the treatment my intent is to create a play/fantasy atmosphere. I often introduce children to the various characters who populate my office. "Fluffy" is a sheepdog doll who lives high on one of my bookshelves; "Lady," a decorative female doll, stands on another shelf near several large prints; and "Longlegs," a goat-like creature with skinny legs, nibbles in the forest of 15 plants that reside on a 30-foot window ledge.

I make these introductions to concretely encourage the child's move from strict reality and to allow her to introduce her own play/fantasy life. Thus, I encourage the "letting go" that helps therapists and patients move to the preconscious and unconscious parts of the mind.

In the first postevaluation session, after Margaret is introduced to Longlegs, she begins to roll some clay aimlessly into a snake-like form. After a few minutes, when I ask her whether she is indeed making another snake (referring to the snake in the evaluation), she informs me that it is a hotdog, and is now actively making a bun to surround the hotdog. Does she need mustard or relish? I ask. She has me make these additional ingredients and then tells me that the hotdog is no good, the bun is no good, and that the mustard and relish are spoiled. I note with a smile that I hear that sometimes Margaret doesn't like to eat too much. Margaret tells me that she *hates* her mother's meat loaf. She had to eat it last night, and her mother didn't let her leave the table until she ate 20 bites, and, she adds, there are a lot of things she doesn't like to eat, and her mother is a bad cook. For example, one day recently she took spaghetti-o's out of a can and that was the whole supper. So, I comment, her mother seems to be a "bad feeder."

Margaret spontaneously tells me about a scary dream she had, and maybe it came from watching a TV episode of *Little House on the Prairie*. It was Halloween. Margaret's family was sitting down, and the lady at the table had no head. She visibly shuddered when she told me about this upsetting scene, and I said, "It must be very scary when thoughts like this come up in dreams."

Margaret notes that every winter she really gets bad dreams. She dreams of hunters and wolves. These hunters come and kidnap her mother and change her into a witch. Then the hunters and wolves go after her. She hopes she won't get these dreams anymore.

I note how upsetting her dreams seem to be, and recall that we have discussed some of her upsetting dreams previously. I discuss why we have dreams—it is as though at night we are trying to figure out some very important things in our lives that are hard to think about during the day. I can see that at night she is doing a lot of thinking, and her mother is very much on her mind.

Margaret noted that she often can't fall asleep at night, that it takes her a long time to get comfortable. When she can't fall asleep, she has a hard time getting up in the morning. She worries that she will be tired and will get a bad grade at school. She hates getting a bad grade. I comment that she usually gets pretty good grades, but that doesn't usually stop people from worrying a lot about any possibility of getting a bad one or even making one mistake. As I speak, Margaret nods her head vigorously about my observation.

The treatment process allows a number of important themes to emerge during this first treatment session: a troubled relationship with her mother, her food aversions related to her mother, her night anxieties and dreams, and her problem with being perfect. I have an opportunity to make these themes explicit to her. It makes it much easier for a therapist to identify themes and have a perspective on their importance if he or she has an assessment workup as a backdrop.

In this session I was struck by how quickly available were Margaret's troubled feelings about her mother. It signaled to me that she was clearly conscious of the fighting parent–child interplay, so I quickly work with her on this issue. Margaret is not aware of the extent of the rage she feels toward her mother: that she sees her mother as a witch, or that the beheaded lady at the table whom she has decapitated in her Little House on the Prairie *dream represents her mother. An eventual goal will be to help Margaret become aware and feel this primitive rage, which is now a forbidden feeling for her.*

Margaret shows some mature motivation for treatment and for working with a "worry doctor." She brings her nighttime worries to the treatment with the implicit wish to have these upsetting feelings taken away.

I also have an opportunity to begin to explore Margaret's problem with being perfect by noting that people can worry about making even one mistake. I will search to develop a metaphor for this problem, such as "She needs to be Miss Perfect." Making this explicit to the patient's ego is the first step in helping her grow to understand why she is driven to be "Miss Perfect." Later, I will add that someone who needs to be perfect on the outside is worried that there is something really wrong on the inside.

After several weeks, Margaret seems to take some proprietary actions. Items on the large, round formica table we sit at—crayons, clay, markers, paper—have been left somewhat strewn about by the last patient. Margaret begins housekeeping, making neat piles, separating broken crayons from intact ones, suggesting benignly by her action that I tend to let things go. She enjoys the domestic role and later initiates all hours by cleaning things up.

In a good mood, she tells me she has had two dreams since we last met, dreams that had good and bad parts to them. In the first dream she was a movie star dancer playing in a theater on 42nd Street. She tells me she loves to dance and that she is a ballerina and ice skater, and she glides gracefully in my office. But in her dream, as she was dancing, she fell down and broke her leg. She awoke from the dream because she felt pain and was relieved that it was only a dream.

Why would a bad part show up in her thoughts when she was having such a good dream? I wonder. Margaret, of course, has no response, and I comment, "Sometimes girls can feel guilty about wonderful excited feelings they have had." They might even find ways to punish themselves for these feelings. Margaret has no response and turns away from me.

But she goes on to another dream (an association, I feel) about taking a shower. In her dream she is taking a shower in the middle of the night. When she turns on the water, it is very hot and she burns herself. She tells me that about a year ago this really happened. It was her mother's fault, because her mother used the bathroom before her. I comment with some wonder, Gee, why would she be having this dream now? Could it be another inside punishment? We must figure out why Margaret feels such a strong need for punishment.

My initial thoughts about Margaret's domestic activity (straightening up my office) were twofold: Was she showing a need to be very

orderly as part of her perfectionism, and/or was this behavior the be-
ginning of a womanly transference? When, further in the session, she
tells me about her star dancing role and begins to exhibit her grace, I
begin to feel that the oedipal transference feelings are predominant. I
was impressed with Margaret's quick ability to bring her dreams and
feelings into treatment, as there is a signiticant percentage of patients
of this age who take much longer to address this kind of material.

The reader may recall that in my evaluation I noted that much of
Margaret's distress was related to unresolved oedipal conflicts. Part
of her difficulties stemmed from forbidden erotic feelings about her
father. I felt she was beginning to transfer these feelings to this new
male in her life, her therapist. My goal is to let these feelings ripen as
they become strongly expressed in the sessions. Eventually, I can
name these feelings to Margaret. For example, I can say she is show-
ing me special daddy-feelings that girls her age develop, about which
they feel both very good and very bad. One needs to wait until these
feelings are palpable in the hour, so that discussion about them is not
just an intellectual observation but rather something the patient can
feel intensely.

Why do disturbing elements emerge in pleasurable dreams? Mar-
garet is the star dancer but suddenly breaks her leg. She looks for-
ward to a shower but burns herself. My thoughts center on her oedi-
pal conflict. If she experiences a female pleasure, she simultaneously
feels she is doing something forbidden. Having womanly feelings
about her daddy is bad, says her internal conscience. Therefore, she
manages via her superego to find a punishment. Margaret is not
aware of any such connection, and I begin to convey the self-
punishment idea ("inside punishment") in the session.

Margaret begins the next session by using the clay to build a house. I
wonder, I ask her, whether she would tell a story about the house, because her imagination helps us do our work. This story unfolds: A
woman is living alone in the house (she uses the Lego figure of a
woman); a storm emerges, knocks the roof off the house; the woman is
hurt and has to go to the hospital. While the woman is in the hospital,
the house is neglected and is populated by spiders and cobwebs. Margaret has taken several spiders and snakes from the toy drawer to wiggle in
the damaged house. She also tells me she is afraid of spiders, especially
tarantulas that are very furry.

Finally the woman has returned from the hospital, and she looks
very, very old. She looks 70 years old and her face is full of wrinkles.
Margaret explains that the woman is really only 48 years old, but they

did plastic surgery on her in the hospital. To make her look older? I ask. She agrees.

Wow, I say. This reminds me of the story of Snow White or Cinderella. Who is going to be more beautiful—the old queen or the young princess; a bad stepmother or the beautiful daughter? Did Margaret know that when girls grow up they naturally want to be more beautiful than their mothers?

Margaret goes to the window where my plants are arrayed. She finds a "dying flower," a geranium blossom that is well beyond full bloom; she suggests that we make a "plantateria" to take care of the dying flowers. Under her direction we construct a little box out of clay, set the dying flower inside, and add some dirt and water as nutrients. This is done tenderly, and we will check on the flower's condition next session. I comment, Gee, this poor old mother blossom needs a lot of care.

In this session I felt we saw further development of the oedipal triangle, in which the major theme was a young girl's rivalry with her mother. Mother is living alone in a house. Tragedy strikes, her home is destroyed, she is injured and hospitalized and further misused by surgeons in the hospital. Margaret expresses her anger with her mother through displacement—forces of nature and physicians (not Margaret) injure and misuse the woman. Because Margaret has already acknowledged difficulties with her mother, I feel that I can directly comment on this kind of intense rivalry in which the issue is over who is more beautiful—Snow White or the queen, Cinderella or the mean step-mother, and by implication, Margaret or her mother.

Margaret responds to my comments, not in direct words but in the concrete metaphors of childhood. She walks to the plant ledge and finds the dying flower, and her ambivalence asserts itself. She has a need to undo her "angry mother wishes." The "dying mother" flower needs nursing care and so the blossom is placed in the "plantateria"— hospital.

I feel this is a wonderful example of how children work in treatment. Over the years they have built up fewer layers of defenses than adults have and often move more easily in their unconscious life. Moreover, the verbalization we see with adults is not available to children; they often speak in concrete metaphor, which is a preconscious language. Margaret finds a dying blossom in the room as a metaphor for her mother. As child therapists we need to speak in turn. Therefore, it is helpful to have a tangible place, a private drawer to house these concrete ideas, and to develop tangible theme folders to concretely elaborate the major issues of the treatment.

CONTINUING WORK WITH MARGARET AND HER PARENTS

In this phase of work with Margaret, themes from the first month of treatment continue to be elaborated.

A family emerges in our play—mother, father, baby, and daughter. The mother is in the bathroom taking a long shower. She is in the bathroom so long that her skin gets wrinkled. In the meantime the daughter prepares meals, feeds the baby and the father. When the father sees the mother after the shower, he says she looks like a prune. I laugh and note that this reminds me again of the Snow White feelings—how mothers and step-mothers turn into ugly old women. I now develop a new book (using a folder), which I entitle "The Family Book." I write several sentences, about how girls want to be pretty and smarter than their mothers and often ask, "Who is better?"

In a later session, Margaret makes a beautiful ring out of clay—which she has stolen from Queen Isabella. Margaret plays a new character who she calls "Miss Shrimpy." In our game she is taken to police headquarters, where she is interrogated by a stern policeman (the therapist). She wants the play handcuffs put on her during the interrogation and her fingerprints taken using fingerpaints. After Margaret acknowledges her crime, she is put in jail by the policeman for 10 years. Toward the end of the session, I write in The Family Book that girls can feel very bad when they have crooked feelings about their mothers. They want to be more beautiful, and they are jealous about all the things that mothers have—jewelry, dresses, perfume, makeup. All girls have these feelings as they grow up. These bad feelings sometimes give girls very bad dreams. (These entries are not made all at one time. They are said aloud and written in the book while Margaret watches and listens.)

In these hours Margaret's play facilitates further discussion of the oedipal rivalry with her mother, and I have a number of opportunities to make her conscious of her jealous feelings and some of her superego responses (Margaret's felt criminizalation and nighttime punishment dreams).

In many of the sessions of this period Margaret continues with her plantateria play. Dying flowers are removed and placed in the plantateria for special care. Some have the sickness "thermolia." She checks on how they are doing, and I call her the nurse of the plantateria. Her interest begins to shift to all the live plants, finding the buds that will soon blossom, and she suggests that we cut off the dead leaves and throw them away. She talks cooingly to the little growing blossoms. I note how all girls have special family feelings as they grow—someday they would like to have their own little plants and little babies to take care of. In fact, it seems as if Margaret is taking care of the little babies in the office. My last comment threatens Margaret; she moves out of the play, goes to the clock to see how much time is left. For the remaining time in the session she sits stiffly on a chair, facing the clock, waiting for the time to elapse. I comment that maybe my "baby" remark made her feel very nervous.

In her play, I felt that Margaret was bringing back in another form the womanly transference. The office was our home, and she was caring for all our babies. The plant play was expressing the daddy feelings, just as her proprietary cleaning up and arranging had done so earlier. But my attempt to make this more conscious—"that girls like to have little plants and little babies to take care of"— caused some excessive anxiety, and Margaret retreated from the play and became frozen.

The preceding experience touches on the theme of the "art of psychotherapy." How do we know when to begin to make a difficult confrontation or to begin an interpretation? The major internal barometer for making interventions is our quality of empathy. Margaret's resistance of the moment certainly indicated to me that her therapist/father feelings made her quite anxious and that I would have to proceed judiciously. At the same time, I thought that although Margaret retreated, she was not overwhelmed. I did not regret introducing this idea into consciousness despite her flight, but it did alert me to her vulnerability.

All therapists struggle with the timing of an interpretation. We utilize an empathy that is developed from both our knowledge of the patient and our intuition at the moment. Timing is not the only issue; the phrasing of an interpretation is also very important. Metaphors in an acceptable play language can typically advance an intervention that is much better accepted by children. Despite intuition and knowledge, however, all therapists will occasionally err in their tim-

ing, and the patient may temporarily retreat. It is rare that any real damage is done to the essential therapeutic process. In fact, despite the anxiety that the dreaded subject may involve, the therapist will find a new way at a later date to successfully broach the subject.

In this phase of our work, Margaret is preparing for a role in a school play that will be performed in front of all the parents. She knows not only her own part, but literally the words of the all the parts of all the actors. She is afraid that some of the children will make a mistake, which would be very embarrassing. She corrects the other students when they make mistakes during rehearsals. Some of the children get angry with her—she is too bossy—and they tell her that she isn't the teacher. But, she explains to me, that if the play is bad, she will be "too embarrassed." I note with her that this is a good example of her "Miss Perfect" worry.

She recalls some very embarrassing things that have happened to her. One day in class she was answering a subtraction problem on the blackboard in front of everyone, but she thought it was an addition problem. This event happened more than a year ago, but she remembers it vividly. I note that when people have to be perfect every day, they worry deep inside that something is very, very bad and that it can come out at any time. (I felt that Margaret was struggling with a dreaded sense of damage about herself, and that she could "undo" that unconscious dread by being mistake-free on a daily basis. Any small error resonated to this fear of her significant underlying defectiveness that stemmed from the mother–child relationship.

The theme of food is also played out. We make meals out of clay—good foods and bad ones. Margaret hates meat loaf and spinach and loves pizza and peanut butter. She begins to talk freely about her mother's bad food. She complains that many times her mother doesn't cook the food long enough, so it doesn't taste good. Sometimes she is very hungry, and her mother doesn't even begin to make dinner.

Margaret writes a letter to her mother. "Do not, I repeat, DO NOT give me squished sandwiches in my lunch box anymore." She adds, "And I still love you." She adds several bubble gum wrapper jokes as little presents to soften the message. She makes an envelope, and we find a stamp and mail it to her mother. "Sometimes you feel your mother doesn't love you when she makes mistakes in your lunch box," I note. I add, "When girls are young, they feel very strongly that moms who love them feed them well." (For the first time, I introduce a new idea.) I comment that when she was a little girl, her mom had some very strong worries and sometimes found it hard to take care of her. So now, Margaret is very sensitive to any food mistake her mother makes. (The mother had confidence that I would broach this material in a way that Margaret could understand.) In Margaret's presence I begin to write about this idea in the Family Book we constructed together.

During this early phase of treatment with Margaret, we see the unfolding of various themes as they fade in and out: mother/oedipal rivalry, father transference, defense elaboration (perfectionism), oral conflicts expressed through food. The therapist needs to maintain internal flexibility, because the themes and issues of the treatment hour can change rapidly.

In the early work with the parents, they feel that Margaret is happier; she appears to be better in school, and she struggles less with the other children.

The parents report that Margaret still tries to be too close to her father. She asks playfully, "Will you be my husband? Are you getting a divorce? How pretty do you really think I am?" Both parents feel this continues to go on too long. Her mother reports that she still gets very irritated with Margaret when she hears these comments. She notes that when she and her husband discuss anything, Margaret is right there to break up the twosome. In my exploration of these incidents, it becomes clear that the mother is still the one to tell Margaret that they are discussing something private, and that she will have to wait. When I wonder with her father why *he* does not tend to shoo Margaret away at these times, he seems puzzled. He says, "I really don't know. I see what you both mean, and maybe I identify with her too much." I wonder aloud whether the father still feels that his wife comes down too hard on Margaret. He nods, and says that he is the one who can always get her to calm down and become reasonable. The mother notes with exasperation, "The problem is that I am always the heavy disciplinarian and he is always the good, reasonable father."

This kind of early discussion of the good-parent, bad-parent split helps the parents to become more fully aware of this troubling division. In fact, they both express some astonishment as to how strong this division seems to be, and how their daughter has exploited the division. With this kind of conscious awareness, the father began to be much tougher, reinforcing rules and figuring out how the mother could do pleasurable things with the daughter.

During the latter part of this phase, the mother began to explore retrospectively some of the tenseness she felt with Margaret during her early years. She felt that many things occurred during the pregnancy, birth, and Margaret's early infancy that set a negative tone. During the pregnancy she had a growing feeling that she was unattractive to her husband. She began to feel betrayed and that having Margaret was a huge burden. In fact, she said, she was indeed actually being betrayed, because her husband had begun his affair during her pregnancy. During the delivery she "lost it" in relation to her husband. She went into a "paranoid state" and wanted him out of the room. She remembered screaming, "Get that man out of the room—he is going to hurt me." During Margaret's infancy there were ongoing troubled feelings. She felt she wasn't an asset to Margaret and that someone else could raise her better. There was a constant question, "Should I be Margaret's mother?" Retrospectively, she now realized that she was feeling that her husband was attached to someone else and that he would rather have that person as Margaret's mother than herself. This material was brought forth with a great deal of anguish, and both parents felt very pained as it was discussed. Simultaneously, it seemed to be providing the mother with some relief and understanding of the trouble in her relationship. I commented that I felt this was very important material. She has always been in a great deal of pain about her feelings of alienation toward Margaret. It seemed to me that she was beginning to describe a very understandable context for how these feelings emerged.

In this phase of work there is an important shift. The reasons for the contamination of the mother–child relationship begin to emerge. Margaret's birth was linked with a traumatic family period. The mother's estrangement from her child reflected her father's estrangement from his wife, both as a husband and the father of her child. This new knowledge and understanding begins to help the mother feel less like a hateful and cruel person as it provides her with a perspective for her feelings of withdrawal from her child.

This kind of work is on another level and involves the techniques of "treatment of the parent–child relationship." (See Part II). The mother seeks to repair her relationship with her daughter and wants help in understanding the unconscious barriers that impede their tie. Although this work involves uncovering important past unconscious factors, it still remains within the domain of parent work. Many child therapists would refer this mother for individual therapy under these circumstances. I feel this would be an unfortunate error. The child therapist has an opportunity to focus on this issue and simultaneously to limit the domain of this work to the parent–child relationship. The child therapist can deal with these issues in a timely manner necessary for Margaret's developmental needs. If I observed, for example, that the mother could not work this through within a reasonable time, an individual referral would be appropriate.

As the early history of Margaret becomes clearer, we can more fully see the dimensions of a significant "developmental interference." (See Nagera, 1966.) The mother's prolonged discomfort with her offspring shaped an internally troubled sense of self in Margaret.

CENTRAL ISSUES WITH MARGARET AND HER PARENTS

In this next phase of the therapy with Margaret, she explores a number of themes related to her early relationship with her mother.

Margaret's play drifts to the paints and finger paints. She discovers a pleasure of messing, the pleasure we describe as "smuching." Colors run all over the white tabletop. In fact, she and I develop a regular "smuch time," which she thoroughly enjoys, and later, at the end of the hour, she works hard to clean up perfectly. She makes a number of comments about how her brother Seth can make a big mess when he eats. Food is everywhere as he learns to feed himself. I am able to note that Seth seems to enjoy the "smuch time" with his mom, but this is something she missed and couldn't have when she was little.

This was unusual play for Margaret because it had a strong regressive quality that was not in keeping with her typical style. My intuitive response was that this kind of "letting go" didn't occur during Margaret's early years because of the internal anxiety and tension of the mother. The new relaxed mother could allow this typical messy play with her second child. The mother felt guilty as she made these comparisons.

The paints now have water added to them, and they become concoctions; these mixtures have glue and sugar added to them. They are placed in plastic milk bottles with nipples on the tops. They gather some sinister features inasmuch as they are made in our special "laboratory"—they become poisons.

Fluffy and Longlegs develop a special baby-sitting service. Armed with this secret milk, they advertise (make little signs), promoting a high-level baby-sitting service that has an international reputation. Parents call the service, and the sitters take their little children on an excursion to the park. Fluffy carries these children and infants on her back, bouncing them along. Of course, the children get thirsty, and they are fed the excellent brew. They quickly die. The mother (another doll figure) comes to pick up her little offspring, and she is told that they are asleep at the bottom of the hill. As the mother goes to wake up her little children, Fluffy and Longlegs push a huge boulder onto the family. Margaret often sings out during the period, "It's baby killing time," and the game ensues.

I make further entries into the Family Book. All older sisters hate their younger brothers, get strong jealous feelings and killing wishes; the killing wishes come up about the mother as well. Margaret has a big, delighted smile whenever she can call out, "It's baby killing time."

I think that this opportunity to play out these intense feelings allows Margaret to feel considerably less guilt and to understand the normal human origins for these feelings.

Despite the rage toward the baby at home, the "babies" in my office are treated differently. The womanly transference noted earlier is expressed in Margaret's care for my plants. These plants become very important to her. She now carefully waters the plants, making sure not to overwater them. She looks closely at the buds and watches the process of "hatching." She looks at the state of each leaf, cutting off the dried ones to keep the plants healthy. Although earlier I emphasized the oedipal nature of the activity, she is now much more focused on maternal care. I feel that each plant is like her baby, and she enjoys providing the best care for each one. In fact, my plants never looked so healthy and green. This watchful activity was done with intense investment.

I comment on what a wonderful mother Margaret had become. I tell her that I know her mother wanted to give her special care when she was little, but many times during those years her mother had many worries and was very upset. When mothers are like that, it's often hard to know what their little ones are feeling. Margaret does make a few comments. She doesn't remember when she was a baby, but she does know that her mom was always upset and fighting with her dad. I comment, "It must be hard to see the special care that Mom now can give to Seth."

As I came to understand this material, I began to feel that Margaret was taking an important turn. She was clearly providing the babies in the office with what she unconsciously felt she hadn't received herself. I felt that this material was coming into the treatment hour because she was witnessing at home a very different mother–child interaction between Seth and her mother. Although Margaret could express her jealous rage in play (the baby-sitting service) she was developing a new capacity. She would overcome the past deprivation by becoming the good mother herself, providing amply for the babies in the office. This was an important passive-into-active mechanism, and I felt it had the potential to be an extremely adaptive behavior. I have often found in treatment that the therapeutic atmosphere allows patients to rework past situations of stress and to begin to find more benign solutions. Margaret's earlier attempt to cope with the frustration was to become the angry attacker. Now she seemed empowered to undo the past by becoming the good, empathic mother herself.

Margaret also makes several multimedia paintings during this period. These paintings are very vivid. They take a long time to make, and Margaret tells me they are sad paintings. One painting is of a small tree in a desert. The tree is disfigured and all dried up. The gnarled quality of the roots and branches is expressed through clay projections on the painting. Not a leaf appears on the branches. Margaret tells me angrily that there is no story about this tree—the tree is just dying because it can't get any water. I note that my plants here are very well fed, but maybe when she was a little tree she felt she didn't get enough to drink. I could see sad feelings cloud Margaret's face.

The second "sad" painting is of a flock of birds, a very dark sky, and a distant light tower of an airport. Margaret angrily told me that this time there is a story! The birds are trying to get to the airport to make a plane, but they are always missing the plane—they always come too late. Finally, they have a chance to make the last plane, and they are on time. But a huge black storm comes up and blows them back. In the distance you can see the plane taking off again without them. The birds, I say, were trying to reach the mother ship (Margaret's puts her fingers to her ears). Something always got in the way; maybe it was the black storms that mother had; maybe it was Margaret's black storms that kept the mother ship away. Margaret looks angry, puts her fingers even tighter over her ears, and sits down in front of the clock until the hour is over.

Despite the overt rejection, I feel a greater bond with Margaret after these comments. She breaks out into a short burst of conversation, talking very comfortably about the events of the last few days since we last met. She describes, for example, with affection, what her brother smells like when he's walking around with a full diaper. She muses about her future marriage—she would want to have several children, but only one at a time because they are hard to take care of. She has a sty on her eye. Could I take a close look at it? She knows she shouldn't rub it, and she used to be afraid that a sty would just grow and grow. Her friend Sarah was angry with her and has nicknamed her "Trouble." That used to bother Margaret, but now she calls Sarah "Fat Bubble" because she is fat. These are most relaxed commentaries about the current scene, stated casually to a close confidante. They describe the thoughts of a youngster who seems generally relaxed and very comfortable in the relationship.

In the parents' session in this period, Mrs. M particularly continues her work on the troubled past marital tension and its implications for the relationship with her daughter.

The mother and father recounted that they had recently gotten into a big fight in their preparation for a holiday dinner. The father had failed to remember to buy a dozen eggs that the mother had needed for a recipe. As they described the event, mother acknowledged that she was carrying around lot of rage inside of her. What stimulated these internal and familiar feelings? For 2 weeks prior to the dinner, the father had been working late in his office. The mother had those old feelings—is he really working late again or out with someone? She even called the office several times and found that he was there, where he should be. She began to realize in this period that she was getting increasingly furious, yelling and screaming at Margaret. We all suddenly realized in the session that Mrs. M was reacting to Margaret as though she were her father's mistress—the other love. This was a very powerful insight for mother. It was such a familiar feeling—a feeling she has been carrying for such a long time, perhaps even before Margaret was born. She cried as she understood what a bizarre idea this was, and what a barrier it had been to her feelings toward her child. In this period she wanted several extra parent appointments to retrace how this idea had expressed itself with Margaret over the years. (Her husband attended all these sessions.) She brought in a locket in which she carried a lock of Margaret's baby hair. She constantly fondled the hair as she spoke, wanting somehow to bring about a close mother–daughter connection. She repeated often in this period, "I know my husband really loves me and Margaret is really my child, but it's been so hard to alter these feelings in the past."
There was little doubt that these new awarenesses began to shift the unconscious ties between mother and daughter. Mrs. M describes how she is doing more fun things with Margaret while her father has more of the chores. Recently, mother and daughter went ice skating together, and the mother felt they had a really good time—a lot of smiles were exchanged as they skated hard, holding hands. When they got home, the

"old Margaret" appeared for a few moments. She made a point of saying to her father in front of her mother, "Why didn't you come? It was no fun without you." Mother described how furious she would have been in the past, but instead she commented playfully that Margaret was trying to make dad feel better because she has the best times with Mother. Margaret broke into a big smile.

The parents reported that the anger that Margaret typically expressed seemed to be receding. Mother and daughter bought a guinea pig together, which Margaret had wanted for a long time. She took instructions from her mother very seriously on the care and feeding of the new pet. They named her "Squeaky" together, and Margaret said a number of times, "I can't believe Squeaky is really mine." Margaret began to try new foods: baked potato, different kinds of eggs that her mother prepared. Her mother now teases her, "Will my pancakes taste as good as Dad's?" Margaret answers playfully, "Never."

Margaret wiggles less at the table and makes no trips to the bathroom while they eat. She actually now works with her mother on what will go into her lunch box, and her mother is allowed to put in a surprise. Recently they have begun to cook together—for example, her mother bakes the cake and Margaret decorates it with icing. The mother clearly experiences an enormous happiness as she can now pleasurably feed her daughter.

I was struck in this period by how critical the work with the mother was in order to alter the mother–child relationship. Despite the intensity of the uncovering work with Mrs. M, it differs in some significant ways from an individual psychotherapy where the mother would be the primary patient. There was a very important underlying boundary—our work centered on the mother–child relationship, and the purpose was to emotionally reunite the estranged pair. Mrs. M clearly did not want to explore other aspects of her life except as they referred to this central theme. Margaret remained my primary patient. It is important to note that a therapist can do intense uncovering work with parents within the domain of "parent work," as long as the goals and boundaries remain clear.

THE TERMINATION PERIOD

The parents described changes in Margaret that seemed to be sustained over several months. Mrs. M and Margaret continued to get on very well. Margaret was eating better, was much more comfortable about food, and there were few flashes of anger expressed toward her mother. The parents were quite impressed by her shifts in peer relationships; they saw much less of her bossiness, and she had clearly developed a best friends group. These sustained changes ushered in a termination period. In this period, Margaret developed a new kind of play.

Margaret developed a blueprint and built a boat, utilizing her multimedia ingredients. She used Legos as the foundation; she added paper clips, clay, cardboard cutouts, and yarn to create her accessories. Slowly, an impressive craft emerged. This was a vast project; it had a main steering and motor section, living quarters with sleeping and eating areas, a hold for storage and supplies, separate lifeboats secured to the main ship, lighting for night travel, and life jackets. It was built, repaired, serviced, and sailed by a 15-year-old girl and her two female friends represented by Lego dolls. They wore monkey suits and got grease on themselves as they worked on the mechanics of the boat. The mother, father, and grandfather financed this operation and visited occasionally to marvel at the construction. Later, they completely disappeared.

A large dock area was also constructed. It housed all the supplies the boat needed: fuel, foods, general supplies, replacements for broken equipment.

The three girl companions carried out all the adventures. The major theme of the stories, once the equipment was erected, was the viability of the boat and the viability of the three inhabitants. The boat did not have a major task. There was no fishing; it didn't travel from place to place or deliver goods to a foreign port. Its function was maintenance and self-survival in stormy seas. When the rudder broke down in the ocean, the girl mechanics swam under the boat to repair the damage. When the food supply was low, one of the girls fished from a lifeboat. She was separated from the main craft by sudden waves but was rescued by a radio system housed on the lifeboat and connected to the main cabin.

Many sessions were spent on the long "lifelines" leading from the dock, which could be attached to similar lifelines on the boat (long strands made out of clay). These lifelines were like hoses, and the ends could be fit together. Resupply regularly occurred when the hoses were connected, and supplies were suctioned from the dock to the ship's hold.

This was very intense and pleasurable play. Because of the stormy sea, the ship often could not dock. At times when the hose connection was made, the sea ripped it apart. The teenage divers needed to swim underwater to repair the damage, and it was touch and go as to whether the supplies would eventually be delivered. It was interesting to note that while the boat was on the ocean, it never strayed very far; it stayed within the proximity of the supply dock. The lifelines were often cut and repaired; damage was done by sea currents and other boats, and on one occasion by the teeth of a shark. Despite all these disruptions, the strength and ingenuity of the female repairers won out.

After the ship was finally resupplied, the weary girls went to the living area. They cooked a huge meal—spaghetti and meatballs, cake and ice cream—to replenish their energy.

I found this ongoing story to be a very interesting review and reworking of some of the major themes of the therapy. I felt that the boat was the symbol for the mother ship that sustained life at sea. It was the resurrection of the mother who sustained life during the child's early years. The captain of the boat and her companions struggled to get the supplies and nurturance. The tension in the story was whether supplies could be cut off and the intensity of the storms (the troubled mother–daughter relationship) the girls would experience. The quest was to be sufficiently fed and nurtured despite the "storms" of the ocean. The supply lines—the umbilical cords—could be severed. I felt that Margaret continued to reexperience the early trauma in her life.

Margaret's boat play and her simultaneous effective functioning at home and school made me feel she had found a useful solution to her internal conflicts. Freud (1914) described the enormous potential for change through work within the therapeutic hour: "Past experience can be rendered harmless by virtue of its admission into the transference as a playground in which it is allowed to expand in almost complete freedom, and in which it is expected to display to us everything in the way of pathogenic instincts that is hidden in the patient's mind."

During the earlier course of treatment, a major theme of starvation and nurturance became critical. Margaret guarded against maternal threat and injury through the "identification with the aggressor" defense. She became angry with the mother who did a poor job with the lunch box. She attacked the mother feeder and other children. Using this mechanism, she warded off feelings of helplessness, and she became the powerful attacker. This was a troubling defense, because it alienated Margaret from her mother and from her peers and teachers. I felt that in the course of her treatment she was able to develop a much more adaptive coping mechanism, which helped her deal with the long-standing threat. Margaret appeared to develop "an identification with the nurturer." The "baby" plants in my office received excellent care from a nurturing Margaret, and this gratifying behavior grew as the therapy proceeded. The boat play utilized a similar coping capacity. The 15-year-old captain moved away from the family, and she herself took on the responsibility for life-sustaining tasks, a self-nurturing. Thus, I felt, Margaret was able to make a very important shift—from coping as an "aggressor" (nonadaptive) to coping as a "nurturer"—and I felt this shift resulted from the therapeutic opportunity. Initially, the therapy opened and exposed the conflict, the patient expressed her long-standing and troubled attempts to cope with the threat, and found through play, exploration, and understanding a new and more adaptive means to manage the past interferences. I also felt that this mechanism was facilitated by the mother's new real ability to nurture her daughter more effectively because of the mother's insights in the parent work.

The boat play not only highlighted Margaret's effective coping but also indicated to me her significant move into latency. The 15-year-old captain moved away from her family (the major parent figures remained on the shore), and she and her companions took on all the life-sustaining tasks. This behavior mirrored Margaret's reality separation from her parents and the earlier problematic triangulation of the oedipal period. Her investment was in these new peers, her best friends group. This represented an appropriate shift in latency from the libidinal center of the family to a new center in the outside world.

With sustained good functioning over several months in this last phase, the decision was made to terminate the 15-month treatment.

BIBLIOGRAPHY

Freud, A. (1960). Identification with the aggressor. In *The Ego and the Mechanisms of Defense*, pp. 117–131. New York: International Universities Press.

Freud, S. (1905). *Three Essays on Sexuality* (Standard Ed., Vol. 7). London: Hogarth Press.

Freud, S. (1914). *Remembering, Repeating and Working Through* (Standard Ed., Vol. 12). London: Hogarth Press.

Freud, S. (1924). *The Dissolution of the Oedipus Complex* (Standard Ed., Vol. 19). London: Hogarth Press.

Gross, G., & Rubin I. (1972). Sublimation. *Psychoanalytic Study of the Child* 27:334–359. New York: Quadrangle Books.

Nagera, H. (1966). *Early Childhood Disturbances: The Infantile Neurosis and the Adult Disturbances.* New York: International Universities Press.

Nagera, H. (1981). The developmental profile. In *The Developmental Approach to Childhood Psychopathology*, pp. 3–36. New York: Jason Aronson.

Peller, L. (1954). Libidinal phases, ego development and play. *Psychoanalytic Study of the Child* 9:178–198. New York: International Universities Press.

Piaget, J. (1967). *Six Psychological Studies.* New York: Random House.

Sarnoff, C. (1976). *Latency.* New York: Jason Aronson.

Shapiro, T., & Perry, R. (1976). Latency revisited. *Psychoanalytic Study of the Child* 31:79–105. New Haven: Yale University Press.

Tyson, P., & Tyson, R. (1990a). Psychosexuality. In *Psychoanalytic Theories of Development*, pp. 41–68. New Haven: Yale University Press.

Tyson, P., & Tyson, R. (1990b). The development of the ego. In *Psychoanalytic Theories of Development*, pp. 295–320. New Haven: Yale University Press.

Tyson, P., & Tyson, R. (1990c). The superego. In *Psychoanalytic Theories of Development*, pp. 195–240. New Haven: Yale University Press.

Index